Because I'd Hate to Just Disappear

D1571271

BECAUSE I'D HATE TO JUST DISAPPEAR

My Cancer, My Self, Our Story

Don Hardy, with Heather Hardy

UNIVERSITY OF NEVADA PRESS *Reno & Las Vegas*

University of Nevada Press | Reno, Nevada 89557 USA
www.unpress.nevada.edu
Copyright © 2018 by University of Nevada Press
All rights reserved
Cover photograph by Stacy Burton
Cover design by TG Design

LIBRARY OF CONGRESS CATALOGING-IN-PUBLICATION DATA
Names: Hardy, Donald E., 1955- author. | Hardy, Heather K. (Heather Kay), 1952- author.
Title: Because I'd hate to just disappear : my cancer, my self, our story / by Donald E. Hardy
    with Heather K. Hardy.
Description: Reno : University of Nevada Press, [2018] | Includes bibliographical references.
Identifiers: LCCN 2017038041 (print) | LCCN 2017040997 (e-book) | ISBN 978-1-943859-73-3
    (paperback : alk. paper) | ISBN 978-1-943859-76-4 (e-book)
Subjects: LCSH: Hardy, Donald E., 1955- —Health. | Leukemia—Patients—United States—Biog-
    raphy. | Linguists—United States—Biography.
Classification: LCC RC643 .H29145 2018 (print) | LCC RC643 (e-book) | DDC 616.99/4190092 [B]
    —dc23
LC record available at https://lccn.loc.gov/2017038041

The paper used in this book meets the requirements of American National Standard for Information Sciences—Permanence of Paper for Printed Library Materials, ANSI/NISO Z39.48-1992
(R2002).

FIRST PRINTING

Manufactured in the United States of America

Contents

Contents

Preface

July 2016

THIS IS A COLLABORATIVE EFFORT: most of the account comes from my pen but features responses to each chapter from Heather, my wife. I wrote a little over half of my part of the book after I was diagnosed with leukemia and lymphoma and during treatment. As I remember my original intention, I wrote to relieve anxiety and to record my thoughts during a sequence of experiences that I never, ever imagined I would undergo. Although I had always thought that I was a pessimist, pessimism, I now think, is a pale and weak philosophy that should tremble in the vast shadow of fate. "The worst" became and remains unimaginable. Even after the experiences narrated in this book, I believe that I am an extraordinarily lucky man, but experience has humbled my imagination. Never again will I pretend I can anticipate the "worst" or "best" that the future might bring in harsh revelation. So the first half of this book relates the experience of what was for me the previously unimaginable terror of diagnosis and then treatment for non-Hodgkin lymphoma. Before and during treatment I was for the most part quite literally too scared and sick to engage in much introspection. As the narrative progresses, if it should appear that my writing becomes more thoughtful and introspective, it is because that progression from pre-diagnosed naïveté to post-treatment introspection is my lived experience. I am the chief buffoon-philosopher you'll get to know in these pages.

The experience was raw because it felt as though my life was stripped to the hard bone, as I almost literally was because of the alarming amount of weight I had lost before diagnosis. That the book you hold in your hands contains not just raw experience but also a good deal of humor, goodwill, and introspection is a testament to the kindness that surrounded and sustained me during days when, honestly, I felt it would have been easier to die than to suffer anymore. Take this book primarily as the record of one who at least thinks he now knows more about the gratitude that can come from being forced by fate to recognize the fearful gift of mortality.

Memoirs are among the most intimate of literary genres, but they can invite criticism in some unexpected ways. I felt that I had represented Heather, my wife, relatively well in early chapters, but when I shared my work with friends whom I trust and who know us both, several said that Heather's voice needed to be stronger, more prominent, or maybe even that she needed to write her own account of our experiences. Even then I thought my portrayal of Heather's voice was strong enough, possibly because of my close proximity to the source. But finally I was persuaded to include Heather's voice more prominently in this final version because she herself complained that when I represented her voice, I was doing it wrong. "I don't sound like that. In this chapter you make me sound like you. I would never say that," she would say. I countered with, "Heather, that's why it's called a memoir. That's how I remember you or how I remember you said something." She said, "Well, you remember wrong, as usual." I bargained: "You can edit anything out or change or add anything that you don't like," but that idea held no force with her at all.

Maybe I should explain here that Heather and I are both linguists, so we enjoy arguing about language and spend a lot of time doing it. Heather, though, has spent much of the last thirteen years of her academic life as a dean, probably having to argue about most things.

Anyway, I realized that this "editing" solution might solve Heather's problem with my misrepresenting her voice, but it wouldn't increase the representation of her views that my readers were suggesting. So I offered another deal: "Okay, you get to edit or change anything you want, and I think it would be great if you wrote five-hundred-word rejoinders to each chapter. The responses can be longer or shorter if you want, but around five hundred words would probably be ideal."

Heather enthusiastically agreed. And the more I thought about it, the more I realized that including Heather's original voice in the book would make it more fun. I was right about this, if nothing else. She is an excellent writer, and she's very, very funny. Not as funny as I am, of course, but that's a private argument. And I strongly believe that sharing this project, in addition to sharing the responsibility for keeping me alive, has brought us closer together. I, for instance, now have a greater appreciation for her humor, her outstanding editorial and organizational skills, and her attention to detail. It is, I think, no exaggeration to say that both literally and figuratively she has saved my life.

The book is written in a strange genre that no one so far as I know has figured out. It is creative nonfiction, Heather tells me, which almost sounds like a good category. The point is that a good number of things in the book happened, or mostly happened, as I describe them. And when I get things wrong, which is a central trope of the story, Heather comes in behind me to set the story straight. We've talked over almost every event narrated in the book between ourselves and sometimes with others. I don't identify the people I talk about by real name or by any name other than for Heather and me (and those that appear in research references and acknowledgments). I have tried to represent my increasing awareness or knowledge as I experienced it, in real time. When I am found to be wrong, I point that out later in the book, or when research or treatment has changed from the way I present it early on, I correct that later, corresponding with when I discovered the new information. One important caveat to offer is that it is nearly impossible to stay on top of developments in research and treatment relevant to my health unless you are an oncologist specializing in my particular cancer. And, even more important, I need to explain that I have a medical excuse for the inaccuracy of some of my account during treatment—the confusion caused by chemo fog, in which it is difficult to remember accurately, or sometimes even at all. Mental confusion and the resulting anxiety are inevitable and absolutely indispensable parts of the story of my experience with chemotherapy. Those experiences are commonly reported in current research, well known to people who have been, as I like to say, "cooked." Although I've scrupulously tried to be accurate about the medical details of my treatment and condition, I can almost guarantee you that I've gotten some things wrong, simply because I am not an oncologist. I don't want to get all metafictional, but isn't some fiction partially fact and some fact partially fiction? If these categories—fact and fiction—didn't leak into one another a little bit at times, in the real world or at least in the reader's mind, I couldn't imagine wanting to read either. Human desire, what we want or think we want, what we need or think we need, seems essential to both.

After I'd finished a final draft of this manuscript, I read a book that had been suggested to me as relevant to my interests: Stewart Alsop's *Stay of Execution: A Sort of Memoir*. I'm taking a moment here to recommend it myself because it is a beautiful book, written in a different time in American politics, history, and cancer treatment (the early 1970s). Alsop's memoir reminds me of how lucky I am, why any of us attempt to write, and how I've tried to be honest here, whether I've succeeded or not.

Because I'd Hate to Just Disappear

Not a Clue

July 24

I DIDN'T EVEN KNOW enough to suspect.

I've had high white blood cell counts at least since the second of my two shoulder surgeries when I was in my fifties. My literally tall, dark, and handsome orthopedic surgeon said, "Hey, you have a slightly elevated white blood cell count, but we're going to go ahead and operate." I said, "Okay, is that because of the inflammation in the shoulder?" He said, "No, it could be any number of things," a sentence that, while undeniably true, I've come to distrust because I've also learned that it gives me permission to search for any excuse not to make eye contact with serious illness.

When I'd thought about cancer in my life, which was infrequent, I thought mostly about lung cancer because I had smoked for a number of years. I quit thirty years ago and have never been tempted since. Any of the other forms of cancer—pancreatic, liver, skin—I dumped in the same risk category as airline accidents or being hit by a meteor—too unlikely to think about seriously. I mistakenly thought leukemia was a childhood disease, and I had already survived childhood, the worst of the medical part of it being chronic asthma, which is only one reason I frequently congratulated myself on quitting smoking when I did. So I immediately filed the high white blood cell count in my mental recycling bin.

I had vaguely suspected the onset of the first of my two bouts with adhesive capsulitis when I could no longer raise my left arm for balance in playing racquetball or even take a glancing blow off the left court wall without agonizing pain. For whatever reason, some folks develop scar tissue in the shoulder joint that tightly binds the joint and prevents movement without pain. As the pain gets worse and worse, one naturally restricts movement in that shoulder more and more, which in turn encourages the growth of additional scar tissue.

I had been noticing restricted motion and increasingly greater pain in my left shoulder, the first to freeze up, when I reached to pull the overhead screen down in my classroom or sometimes when riding my motorcycle, with my arms extended relatively straight. I unconsciously took to riding with only one hand, my right, on the handlebars because of the pain in the left shoulder.

After the surgery, I got on with my months of physical therapy accompanied by the second of my strictly controlled experiences with oxycodone. If you have intense shoulder pain from adhesive capsulitis (colloquially known as "frozen shoulder") or a torn labrum, there are very good reasons to just go ahead and have the surgery, in my experience: although the post-operative pain will, for a while, be very bad, the surgery will most likely be the first step to ridding yourself of the intense pain and heavily restricted motion in your shoulder. One danger of any surgery of this sort, however, is that the post-operative pain must frequently be controlled by opioids, in the case of my shoulder surgeries, mainly oxycodone—what has become for many poor souls either a gateway drug to heroin or an addiction in itself that has led to misery, wrecked lives, and even death.[1]

I've read that it is extraordinarily easy to get hooked on oxy. Just yesterday a local pharmacy, not the one that I use but the one closest to my house, was robbed at gunpoint, not of money but of drugs. Details haven't hit the paper yet, but I'd bet money that the gunmen made off with a large plastic bottle of oxycodone—sometimes called hillbilly heroin. Oxycodone, along with all the other narcotics that patients in chronic pain are lucky to have access to, is a dangerous drug, but if you're under the care of a physician who respects pain and the dangers and benefits of narcotics, and if you can resist the urge to lose control with oxy, the drug makes bearable not only the immediate post-operative pain of shoulder surgery but also the suffering involved in the weeks of necessary physical therapy. If you didn't have the oxy, you might very well try to gouge out the eyes of your physical therapists to stop them from pulling and scraping bones on bones bristling with newly inflamed nerves in your shoulder joint.

In all of my experiences with oxycodone, when I no longer needed the drug for pain, I deliberately tapered off my usage so that I was at the end down to no tablets at all. I missed the mood boost for about two days, but I didn't suffer withdrawal or any other negative psychological effects. As you will see throughout this book, I have been extraordinarily lucky with all my experiences with medically required opioids, somehow avoiding the common and tragic road of addiction. On reflection, opioid addiction is one of the horrible fates that I am most grateful that I was spared.

At physical therapy they called me Sunshine. Occasionally I brought the staff coffee and donuts. I suspect I'm not the only one who experienced transference of some sort with the staff since I regularly spied pin-pupiled grinning patients bringing in casseroles and lasagnas. Nonetheless, to a person, the physical therapists were fit and full of boundless energy.

But back to my handsome doctor's office. "Hey, you have a slightly elevated white blood cell count" should have sent me screaming to the Internet. If you simply google "high white blood cell count," one of the first hits is for a website at mayoclinic.org. Now, the truth is the Mayo Clinic treats a detailed list of disorders, including dandruff and delayed ejaculation, but if you say, "Mayo Clinic," I say, "Cancer." I know jack about medicine, which is the first and most important reason you should trust nothing I say in this book about medicine or cancer or treatment or doctors or surgeons or even band-aids. The other reason to trust nothing here is that this book is crawling with deliberate omissions and slight distortions (both only to protect the innocent), much as my blood is crawling with whiny little do-nothing cancerous cloned white blood cells that are equally invisible to the unaided eye. (I've never been warned not to anthropomorphize my cancer cells. It's my minor revenge on them.) My omissions and distortions, however, have no real effect on the robustness or reliability of the narrative.

So fast-forward a year to a routine blood test showing even higher elevations of white blood cells (oh, around 13,000 while normal counts are "4,500-11,000 white blood cells per microliter (mcL)").[2] This time I pointed out to a physician's assistant that I had swollen lymph nodes in my neck. Yep, you guessed the answer: "That could be any number of things," which remained as true as the first time. The physician's assistant did say that we would be looking into the possibility of leukemia if the white blood cell count went extraordinarily high. If you google "swollen lymph nodes and high white blood cell count," among the first hits is www.webmd.com/cancer/understanding-leukemia-symptoms. It seemed impossible to me that I could have leukemia, what I now realize was a foolish impression unintentionally reinforced by the youthful optimism of the physician's assistant, who probably quite rightly did not want to send me in a panic to Google over a false scare.

Did I google the phrase? No. Did I follow up on the recommended blood test six months later? No. Am I an idiot? Yes. Did I make a fatal mistake? No. Was I extraordinarily lucky? Yes. I have CLL/SLL, as chronic lymphocytic leukemia and small lymphocytic lymphoma are known among the cognoscenti. CLL/SLL frequently but not always takes its own sweet time killing its victims. If I had acute lymphocytic leukemia, which as I understand it is much more aggressive than CLL/SLL, I would not be referring to myself as lucky.[3]

I did have the blood test over a year later. By then, my white blood cell counts were around 48,000, and I had more swollen lymph nodes. Yet after even more blood tests (details to follow later) and a lymph node biopsy confirmed CLL/SLL, my oncologist, whose every syllable I hang on, said I was in the "watch and wait" mode, meaning no treatment at that time. So even though I don't recommend my brand of idiocy to anyone, my burying my head in the sand might have bought me six relatively stress-free months of ignorance, if not bliss. I honestly don't know whether I now appreciate those six months or not, because having cancer has changed me, I hope for the better, in many ways. But the change wasn't and isn't easy. The mix includes fear, pain, fatigue worse than I could have possibly imagined, mental confusion, derailed work, stress, and life-attitude adjustments that I also couldn't have imagined outside a work of fiction six months earlier.

I should have at least suspected. Two of the symptoms of CLL/SLL are fatigue and "unexplained weight loss."[4] The unusual fatigue had been with me for a couple of years, and it was getting worse. I would teach a class at my university and have to go back to my office, close the door, put my feet up, and take a fifteen-minute nap to recover. Teaching exhausted me. But teaching is always tiring, and I was getting older, so wasn't it natural to be more worn out? And I wasn't always tired enough to have to take a nap after every class. It's like balding. I can't name the day that I categorically had male pattern balding, but I've been losing my hair since my twenties. Now, in my late fifties, I have the inverse of a mohawk.

The clearest sign of the cancer was weight loss, but it was easy to explain that because I was eating an almost entirely vegetarian diet. I went from a norm of about 165 pounds to 145 pounds in a couple of years. My pants didn't fit. I had to gouge new holes in my belts. My friends said I looked terrible. They brought me cookies, which I ate. I still lost weight. So I believed my weight loss, while extreme, was not technically unexplained. I thought I was eating healthier meals, which I probably was, at least for the first year, but I was becoming progressively weaker and more fatigued. In the last year I pretty much lost all interest in food. I ate the very same thing every day for dinner: cheese enchiladas with variable quantities and types of vegetables mixed in. I prepared my own dinner every night because I couldn't stand the thought of eating anything other than this bland invention I was fixated on.

Another odd quirk is that I got myself hooked on oatmeal cookies in about the same time period. I told my physician's assistant once, "I think I have a monkey on my back." That got her attention because I'm sure the first thing she thought was that I was hooked on oxycodone or was selling the oxycodone to buy heroin, the latter being a common developmental stage in the life of a junkie, so I've heard. I said, "I eat six to eight oatmeal cookies a night." She looked relieved, and we laughed. She said, "There are worse things. We just need to watch your triglycerides."

Heather blames herself for not recognizing the signs that something was horribly wrong. I am a stubborn person not easily swayed by either rational or emotional arguments. No doctor ever asked about my diet, which seems now to be one of the things that ought to be first on the list of general checkup questions: "What are you eating these days?"

A friend confided to me after my cancer diagnosis that he almost asked me if I had cancer because I "had that look." He should know. Within a year of their marriage his first wife had died of osteosarcoma, which metastasized to her lungs. I doubt he was the only one who wondered about cancer. I have another friend who simply said many times, "You look awful. You've got to eat more." And she would bring me cookies. And I would eat them, and I would gain no weight.

The sign that should have been like a flaming sword cutting through the evening sky was the night that I became so dehydrated that I nearly lost consciousness. I had stayed at work late, after six, to observe a colleague teaching a graduate seminar. As the class progressed, I started craving water so much that I seriously considered grabbing a student's water bottle. University of Nevada, Reno sits in the geographical transition between desert and the western Sierra Nevada mountain range. It is an arid environment, at high altitude as well, about 5,000 feet above sea level. Most students who grew up here lug water bottles with them everywhere. I've never been a big water drinker, probably resulting in chronic dehydration. That evening, as I became weaker and weaker and craved water more and more, I said, "Excuse me" and went into the hallway to the water fountain. I drank and drank and drank, but I couldn't quench my thirst, and I got increasingly weak, to the point that I was on my knees beside the water fountain. I couldn't stand up. When the professor whose class I was observing saw me through the doorway, he gave the class a break and came out into the hall to see whether I needed an ambulance. I said no and called Heather to come get me. I couldn't trust myself to drive.

Everything in my body was screaming that there was something wrong. I was malnourished, chronically dehydrated, fatigued. What did I attribute these changes to? I was finally getting in shape, dammit! I had bought an expensive road bicycle and somehow found the energy to ride it once a week for a couple hours with friends, although I was always at the end of the pack.

And the damnedest thing of all is that not two months before I was diagnosed with cancer, just on the eve of sixty, I had pretty much decided that my life was over anyway. This is the hardest thing to admit. I am ashamed. But the depression I have long suffered from has little logic or pride in itself. One might as well be ashamed of having cancer or heart disease as feel guilty for clinical depression. And it's not as if I wallowed in it, as is sometimes the idiotic stereotype. I haven't drunk alcohol for the past fifteen years, not because I'm an alcoholic, which is the very first thing that many people confidently and sometimes loudly assume, but because I am clinically depressed. Just about the worst thing you can put in your body if you are depressed is alcohol, even though it is not unusual at all for depressed people to counterintuitively self-medicate with alcohol. I think it is the brief, passing feeling of euphoria that depressives who drink are after. What many of us don't want to accept is that there is an inevitable depressive crash that takes us lower than where we started. That's why I quit drinking alcohol. Because it is really bad *for me*.

I was feeling as if my career was at a dead end, that I was stuck in a drowning department, that my college was being left behind in the headlong, mindless rush to support STEM disciplines (science, technology, engineering, mathematics) to the detriment of everything that a liberal education once stood for, and I believed all these irrational things, fears that are no more well reasoned than your average meme on Facebook. I believed that from here on my life was going to be one long, slow decline into old age and irrelevance, the end result of an inevitable obsolescence of the kind of work I did, linguistics. Eleven months later the worst of my depression was under control. Fighting for my life made me value it more.

Until my fifties my major battles were with depression and anxiety. Before my shoulder surgeries, and then the diagnosis of cancer, most of my struggles were mental rather than physical. Once my problems became more physical than psychological, my survival instinct kicked into high gear. Many people I've known who suffered with depression when they were young overcame that disease when they had children. I think survival and purpose are the common threads. It's what I think attracts some people to war and others to physical violence of any sort. Physical pain is almost always preferable to psychic pain. How many times do you hear, "So-and-so just lost a long battle with depression" versus "So-and-so just lost a long battle with cancer"? Linguists have a way of determining the relative frequencies of expressions like this in languages. *The Contemporary Corpus of American English* (coca), which is over 520 million words in length, cites 169 instances of "battle with cancer" but only 11 of "battle with depression." There is not a single example of "battle against depression." For a battle *against* something you apparently need a physical and concrete enemy, as in "battle against cancer" (with 35 examples in COCA) or "battle against terrorism" (with 58 examples in COCA) or even "battle against terror" (with 12 examples in COCA).[5] That *terror*, that most difficult of modern human aberrations to define, is somehow more concretely something to be battled against than depression perhaps reveals something horribly abstract about our fears and horribly neglectful of our real suffering. Depression seems a battle against the self, waged by the self.

Heather Responds to
"Not a Clue"

I did feel horrible. I knew something was wrong: the weight loss, from skinny to haggard guy, the bizarro eating habits, the constant complaint "I feel like an old man." I also remember with guilt feeling pissed off when he would say that because he is, after all, three years younger than I am. When he was diagnosed I also remembered all the times I pushed his fears to the back of my mind.

I instinctively recognize a sick cat or dog right away. Maybe I unconsciously monitor their behavior since they can't talk. I knew that both Sam and Travis were sick before Don did, and we got them to the vet at least in time for the vets to try, unsuccessfully, to save their lives. But humans are harder, especially Don, because I attributed his weight loss, complaining, and odd eating habits to his depression, which I have never fully understood but have gotten better at coping with over time. I was blessed to grow up confident and cheerful in a happy family. Don's family was troubled.

When Don and I were young, in our thirties, I had no clue how to deal with his depression. I finally figured out on my own and had reinforced in therapeutic sessions with Don's psychologist that the best thing is to do nothing and live my own life. I'm not supposed to try to fix Don, as much as I may want to, because it's futile and "not my job." Don's the only person who can fix himself. I'd come to this realization on my own, but the therapist gave me permission not to feel guilty.

The oddest thing to me about Don's depression is that it seems partly a result of his feeling like everything is his responsibility, that if something is wrong, it's his fault. His psychologist has at least convinced his conscious mind that his obsession with self-blame is, paradoxically, wrongheaded. He's told Don, multiple times, that every time he thinks he's made some kind of mistake, especially one of the catastrophic kind, he must tell himself that he's wrong. At one time he had Don so convinced of the fallibility of his self-directed faultfinding that Don's wallpaper on his smart-phone read, simply, *"Wrong!"*

And here I am adopting one of Don's worst mental habits—blaming myself for mistakes I didn't make just because every-thing's not perfect, because my husband was unlucky enough to get cancer. Yeah, I'm a perfectionist. That's one of *my* psychologi-cal issues.

All the studies we've read say that there are no known risk factors for CLL/SLL, at least no risks that Don had in his history, and that catching it early does not improve the odds of survival. Yet I was disturbed in those early weeks with thoughts of how I could possibly have missed what I thought of as the obvious signs of physical illness.

When I confess this concern to Don, he dismisses it, just as he's done whenever I've tried to fix his depression over the years. He tries to cure my misguided need to feel responsible for fixing his problems, just as he always has. Neither one of us has any business practicing psychology, although my line of work seems to require it occasionally. So although I waited too long, I finally insisted that he go see my family physician.

Notes

1. Kounang, "Opioid Addiction Rates Continue to Skyrocket."
2. Chen, "wbc Count."
3. "What Is Chronic Lymphocytic Leukemia?"
4. *Understanding CLL/SLL* (2016), 17.
5. Davies, *The Corpus of Contemporary American English.* There are more sophisticated statistical tests that I could have performed with the coca data, but this is not that kind of book. Luckily for you!

No Matter What It Is

July 27

I GOT MYSELF a new family physician, partly to avoid the embarrassment of going back to my old one and having to explain why I'd been a doofus and not gotten my next six-month blood check. Heather had been wanting me to switch to her family physician for a long time anyway because she *really* likes him and because we normally have the same family physician to make appointments and checkups a bit easier. I'm not really sure why I didn't get the blood test done on time. It's probably that I'm a procrastinator, or that I was afraid of what the tests would show, or that I was busy with work and coping with the fatigue—or, well, I honestly don't know or don't want to know.

I usually like everybody Heather *really* likes. So I make and keep an appointment with the new family physician. The nurse takes my temperature and blood pressure. My blood pressure is high. I tell her that it is unusual for it to be high. She says, "Maybe it's because you're here." I say, "Maybe," thinking in some dark corner of my brain, "Please don't let it be cancer, please!" The nurse goes over my medications with me: the lisinopril (yep), the clonazepam (yep), the venlafaxine (yep), the Benadryl (when needed): all the drugs that I've been taking for many years now, not to cure me of anything but instead to keep the blood pressure, the moods, and the allergies balanced like a Calder mobile. She says, "The doctor will be with you soon."

It's maybe ten minutes before that quiet knock on the door of the examining room, the slight pause, and the entrance of the family physician. I love that respectful knock and the perfectly timed pause. It's completely unnecessary, but all doctors whom I like do it correctly. The ones who don't either leave the door to the examining room open, which allows me to hear far too much information that I shouldn't know about people I don't know, or don't pause after the knock, as if signaling that their time is more valuable than the minutes you've spent waiting for them to finish with another patient. My new family physician is maybe twenty years younger than I am, casually dressed, friendly, balding. He's human; I love him. He says, "So, what brings you to see me?" I say, "Well, I've got high white blood cell counts, and I've noticed just in the last month or so that the lymph nodes in my armpits are swelled up like toads." He palpates the armpit nodes briefly. He says, "Do you have night sweats?" I say, "No, I don't think so." He says, "Have you been running a fever?" "No." "Have you lost weight unexpectedly?" I answer, "Nope," my first lie, but I quickly rationalize that it was not "unexpected," given what I've been eating. If I had shown him a picture of myself from two years ago, he'd think "anorexia" or "cancer." "Do you have a rash or itching anywhere?" "Yes, I've had hivelike itching off and on for a while. I thought it might be because I'd developed an allergy to nuts because I eat on average a can per day. I have food enthusiasms. I'm in the middle of a nut enthusiasm now." He pauses and says, "Well, that could be a lot of things." I think, "This is great! He thinks I'm complicated." I feel that I might be developing a bro-crush.

He does a thorough palpation of the lymph nodes in my neck, my armpits, and above my groin. He sits down on his rolling stool and says, "I think you have cancer, probably lymphoma or leukemia, so I'm going to refer you to an oncologist." I suspect that I might not love him anymore. How can he seem so certain? It could be a lot of things.

I said, "I've been googling my symptoms and read that my symptoms could be due to an infection"—because I had spent an hour or two on research immediately before my appointment so I wouldn't sound like I didn't have a clue. I had been alarmed by what turned up as the first hit on "high white blood cell count, itching, swollen lymph nodes": an informative but understandably alarming website on Hodgkin lymphoma.[1] I was so ignorant that I didn't know, or didn't recognize in my reading, that if I had lymphoma it was probably non-Hodgkin lymphoma—not a good thing. Hodgkin lymphoma generally has a better prognosis than non-Hodgkin lymphoma, and I knew that Hodgkin usually strikes the young rather than the old. But I was just starting my cancer education. Skipping all the hits on lymphomas and leukemias, I had concentrated on hits on disorders that seemed infinitely preferable: infection, mononucleosis, tuberculosis, lupus, Epstein-Barr virus, cat scratch fever. I was a cancer skeptic. I calculated that my chances were good because all of the important symptoms of each of these non-cancer diseases were essentially the same, I thought, so I had a roughly equal chance of ending up falling in one of these six buckets as in the leukemia bucket. And besides, who gets leukemia at my age? I didn't know a single person, or even a single story of a person, with leukemia at my age. My ignorance seems shocking to me now.

My face probably showed my alarm because he broke eye contact, looked to the side a bit, and said, "Or it could be something else, but we'll want to determine whether it's cancer first." I still love him. It's him and me against the oncologist now, I mistakenly but hopefully believe. It's really him and me against the laboratory pathologist, whom I'm surprised to discover later I will never meet. I don't know whether pathologists ever have to deliver diagnoses of cancer and other horrible diseases to patients themselves. I kind of hope not, because if there is anyone you want to be brutally and dispassionately honest it would be your pathologist. I think I'd prefer not to meet that person, just as I would never want to meet the computer that scores my SAT or the computer that calculates my credit score. By the way, there's a fair amount of computer scoring in CBCs (complete blood counts) as well, one of the primary diagnostics that tell you whether the chemotherapy you are undergoing is brutal enough to knock down the cancerous white blood cell count to normal ranges.

He gives me an order for a CBC and a chest X-ray and says that a surgeon's office will be contacting me to set up a lymph node biopsy. I think to ask—but not quite fast enough to actually do it—whether we shouldn't see the CBC and the chest X-ray before we start removing parts of my body for biopsy. This will be my first lesson in how difficult it is to remember to ask all the relevant questions when my amygdala is overwhelmed by panic. I called Heather at work from the parking lot and told her that our family physician suspects very strongly that I have cancer. I sat in my hot truck in the sun in the parking lot with the door propped open with my left knee. She said that we would get through it together. We said, "I love you." She told me to be careful driving. I said I would. That drive would also be my introduction to how much willpower and concentration it takes to drive safely when cortisone is flooding your brain and nervous system.

I drove immediately to the imaging center for the chest X-ray. I did only the speed limit the entire way, double-checked green lights, left plenty of room between me and the car in front, and when possible drove in the right lane of a four-lane road. The technician asked why I was having the X-ray taken. I said, "They think I have cancer," noting to myself how strange it was that I used "they," not "I think I have cancer" or even "My family physician suspects that I have cancer." *They* is the pronoun we use when we haven't a clue: "They control the banks and the monetary supply." Although I have only a vague idea (Federal Reserve) of who controls the banks and the money supply, I knew exactly who thought I had cancer. *One* guy, *one* doctor, *one* family physician who with a sentence or two shoved me into the cancer diagnosis machinery.

The subtlety of my denial inherent in the use of *they* was only the beginning of it. There's nothing like a tentative diagnosis of cancer to concentrate the mind on alternative hypotheses. The fact that he had ordered a chest X-ray indicated to ignorant me that he suspected lung cancer. He probably didn't. He likely wanted to know if any of the lymph nodes in my chest were as swollen as the ones that he could palpate in my neck, armpit, and groin. Grotesquely swollen lymph nodes in the chest can cause strokes as well as heart attacks, I would learn later. That knowledge made me wonder about what other metaphorical grenades were set to go off suddenly without a suspicion on my part.

I drove straight to the lab for the complete blood count as well, when normally I would have procrastinated a good healthy week or two before having such tests done. The technician doesn't ask me why I'm having the blood drawn. I flinch a bit when the needle goes into my vein. The technician says, "I'm sorry." I start crying, trying to hide it. The technician says, "Tough day, huh?" I explained, "Yes, it's just that you didn't hurt me really and you apologized and you were so kind." She gave me tissues and said that I could sit there at her station if I wanted. I said no and thanked her, leaving, afraid that if I had stayed I'd just weep more and practically beg her to tell me that my family physician is wrong. And if she hadn't said that he could be wrong, that would haven been even worse. I'm hoping that my rapidly expanding health team is wrong. All of them, at my back, on my side, but fundamentally and emphatically *wrong*.

I realize then that it's going to be hard to be a Marine about all this. That prediction will be pretty much validated during every treatment and recovery week of chemotherapy.

I called Heather from the parking lot of the lab before I drove home because I had told her I would. She left work early and was home maybe ten minutes after I got there. She and I talked about how it could turn out to be nothing but an infection or any of the other malfunctions I had sifted from the Internet that morning.

Anything but cancer. It was a conversation that I would probably have tried to have with the lab technician but somehow had better sense than to begin. But we said we'd get through it together no matter what it was.

Then began the waiting game for the diagnosis. Today? No, not today. Tomorrow? Okay, surely by Monday. And surely they are wrong.

Heather Responds to
"No Matter What It Is"

Don always assumes the worst. This could be any number of things besides cancer. But I can't talk him into that. We can both be stubborn. When we go round and round like this, we might as well go to our respective corners and wait it out because we're like two punch-drunk fighters trading some well-placed but mostly glancing blows in the middle of the ring, exhausted and longing for the bell.

"But your family physician can't diagnose cancer. You have to see a specialist for that."

"He *told* me in his office that he thought it was cancer."

"But he said it could also be something else."

"Only after I pressured him."

"Don, you are not an oncologist. You can't diagnose yourself any more than the Internet can."

"Okay, you explain why I've lost all this weight, why I've got these swollen lymph nodes, why my white blood cell count is up."

"You told me yourself that it could be an infection or mono. You're around students all the time. A lot of them have mono."

"I'm not making out with them!"

"Okay, we're going to get through this, but we're going to have to stop thinking the worst because it's not useful. If it's cancer, which it probably isn't, we'll deal with it. There are treatments. If it's something else, which it probably is, we'll deal with that too and probably be happy to deal with it."

If Don assumes the worst, I always assume the best. I think that's one reason we're a pretty good team. He's always looking for signs of a tornado while I'm trying to spot the rainbow. He'll always come around to my way of thinking eventually. And that's exactly what happens this time, although it's understandable this time since nobody wants to believe they have cancer.

"I don't want to talk about this anymore. We're not getting anywhere at all. I'll just watch a little TV and take an extra clonazepam tonight, and maybe I'll be able to sleep."

"You have to sleep," I said. "Your mind is going to get even more wound up if you don't."

"Heather, you're not telling me anything I don't already know."

But instead of watching TV or even turning the TV on, he lies down on the couch and Lyle (Lovett) jumps up to stretch out on his legs. Lyle's a thirty-pound cocker spaniel lapdog. Then Lyndon (Baines Johnson), our red tabby, sees his opportunity and hops up on Don's chest and starts purring. Lyndon has the loudest purr of any cat I've ever had. He wakes me up at night sitting on my chest purring until I have to use earplugs. During the day he insists on being as close to Don as possible. He's a rescue, like all the animals around here. But poor Lyndon was first adopted by a dog-loving family that treated him like a dog. They gave him dog toys to play with and kept him in a dog crate at night.

That's Don's theory on why Lyndon loves Don so much. Don loves dogs, and the cat thinks he's a dog. It's a theory. Actually, in my experience, animals know where they're most needed, and I already had *my* cat, (Mirabeau B.) Lamar.

Notes

1. "Hodgkin Lymphoma."

Don't Clone This

SELF-DIAGNOSIS VIA THE INTERNET is well known among rea-sonable people for being a horrible idea, but I really can't see the harm in it. If some body part of mine is not acting right or I get an odd number on a blood test, I almost always arrive to see a physician with a self-diagnosis in hand, like a report card on my intelligence and diligence ready to hang proudly on the fridge. Like the time I was convinced that my high liver enzymes meant that I was dying of liver disease but instead I turned out to have what is known as "sludgy bile." My family physician at that time told me to be prepared for gallstones. No problem. I'm ready.

I was back in to my family physician's office soon for a reading of the CBC and the chest X-ray. As expected, the white blood count was high. The chest X-ray revealed nothing of interest, my family physician said. He continued, "Did you know you had gallstones?"

"What do I do about that?"

"Nothing, unless they start giving you trouble. And believe me, you'll know when they start giving you trouble."

Another two hours of research on the Internet. It's rumored that gallstones cause pain for men that exceeds that of childbirth. I'll be sure to mention that to my female nurses if I ever have to have them removed. Nurses love listening to self-made medical experts, especially men, I'll bet.

Before the Internet I would prowl the medical library shelves for photographs, illustrations, and descriptions of whatever horrible medical malfunction I imagined I had, which over the years has included liver disease, lung cancer, diabetes, skin cancer, heart disease, and lymphoma. My first scare with lymphoma turned out to be a lipoma. My physician assured me that it was harmless and told me to go home and "tell the wife" that I was "good for another 40,000 miles." I'm sure if I had neither library nor Internet, I'd strike up awkward conversations with friends, family, and strangers: "Is *your* urine ever more lemony yellow than just yellow yellow?"

I know with absolute certainty that I'm not the only one who self-diagnoses using the Internet and a healthy imagination. Heather once convinced herself with the help of the Internet that she had rabies from a cat bite (from our dear Travis, whom we adopted after we discovered that he was living in our window well during a brutal northern Illinois winter). Our veterinarians convinced her after long argumentation and their own Internet consultation that her self-diagnosis was probably incorrect since there had not been a case of rabies in Illinois for eleven years, and the last case was transmitted through a bite from a bat, not a cat or a dog. We are both just as likely to pry initial informal human medical advice from our veterinarians because we see our veterinarians far more frequently than any of our own personal scientists.

For whatever reason, probably procrastination, I even put off performing my self-diagnosis until the morning before my appointment with my family physician. I wasn't really worried. I was having a great summer. I had written two articles and mailed them to journals by the middle of June, and I had been trout fishing four times in a local river. My preferential diagnosis for my problems was cat scratch fever because I live with two cats. My second choice was mononucleosis, picked up somehow (I couldn't quite reason this through soundly) from handling my college students' exams and papers. In every set, I figured, there is at least one that has been sneezed on.

What I wasn't prepared for was the fervor that grabbed me

the evening of my family physician's tentative diagnosis. Heather and I had dinner together, talking around and around the possibilities, and then we distracted ourselves with a documentary on Hitler's stunning influence over the German state from 1918 to 1933, because we needed to think about something more evil than cancer. After the documentary I got out my laptop and settled onto the couch to do some serious Internet cancer research. Heather said, "Don't stay up too late, okay?" "I won't," I lied. By the way, this book, not being a guide to medical treatment for cancer or any of the other disorders I describe, contains in the notes more references to Internet sources than to traditionally published sources. The reason for that is that this is a memoir. I'm telling you where I got my information, not where I wish I had gotten my information so that it would appear that I was at least marginally medically educated.

My self-assigned job that evening and what turned into the early morning hours was to gain a rudimentary understanding of leukemia and lymphoma. In a few hours I had read many of the available online introductions to leukemia and lymphoma. I decided that I probably had CLL/SLL because I fit the age profile. CLL/SLL almost always hits those over forty; the average patient's age when diagnosed is seventy-one.[1]

If I had leukemia, I had what seemed to me then an odd but ominous disease that somehow involved ever-increasing numbers of white blood cells that are immature and useless clones of one another. And just as threatening is that all these immature cloning cells don't die within the timespan of a normal non-cancerous cell. So they're like your geek friends who for some reason never, ever leave a party at a socially acceptable time. They're the ones wanting to order pizza at midnight when you are just craving your bed and your dog or your bed and your cat. ("Or your wife!" Heather added on reading the first draft of this chapter.)

I was obsessed by two questions: etiology and prognosis. Many sources on the Internet report that CLL/SLL has no known cause, although other well-respected sources report that there are some causal links or suspicion of causal links between CLL/SLL and exposure to chemicals such as benzene and Agent Orange.[2] I've never worked around industrial solvents, and I missed the Vietnam draft by months. Those same sources report that CLL/SLL is slow growing in many, but not all, cases. It appeared that prognosis could range widely from maybe five years to over twenty-five—a long time to spend searching the Internet.

The possible prognoses seemed to me absurdly variable, and in anticipation of what I thought at the time was the worst, I convinced myself that I probably had at most five years to live, not even long enough to retire from my job properly, considering that my usual estimate for retirement age was when they carried me feet first out of the classroom. Only then did I realize that my prediction could turn out to be accurate after all, although I had imagined that day to be impossibly far in the hazy future. By 2:00 a.m. of the day following my family physician's tentative diagnosis, I was convinced of wildly random estimates of etiology (bad luck) and prognosis (five years at most).

My previous indifference to my survival into my fifties is the most astounding thing about my cancer experience, at least thus far. Somehow, maybe because my dad lived into his nineties and my mother is now in her eighties and relatively healthy, I had no gut realization that I had been extraordinarily lucky to live into my late fifties almost untouched by invasive disease and medical treatment. Now when I hear of someone dying in childhood or as a teenager or as a young adult or even in their forties or early fifties, I think how brutal and arbitrary fate is. All those years I've had that so many other people don't get, and I haven't really appreciated them until now. My dying regret might turn out not to be that I didn't live longer but that I didn't use the years I was gifted with more productively or thoughtfully or lovingly. A future lost might be a past regretted. Of course, now I want to live into my eighties at least, against all odds for someone with CLL/SLL, and I want to use that time as if it were gold flakes I had to measure out to purchase the bare necessities of life: food, rest, shelter, love, thoughtful reflection. No time to waste now. Fewer than twenty-four hours since my family physician had first used the word *cancer*, I was already trying on the gown of sage philosopher.

The truth was I couldn't even intelligently guess at the answers to many of my questions without the results of the blood sample taken the previous day. I wasn't even sure how a final diagnosis would be made. Some resources suggested that a diagnosis could be easily determined by a pathologist examining my blood in the laboratory; others suggested that perhaps a lymph node biopsy (mentioned also by my family physician), or even a bone marrow sample, must be taken and analyzed by a pathologist. Even I recognized by two in the morning that I was stuck in an infinite loop of ignorance and contradictory information.

That's when my friend Jon sent me a friend request on Facebook. With only a second of hesitation (because wasn't Jon already my friend on Facebook?), I accepted the request. It seemed a kind of small miracle. I really needed to talk to a friend about the news, and Jon was perfect. Jon has been through medical hell in his life: at least one shoulder surgery, two hip replacements (the second to replace one that had failed from longevity), knee replacement, left ankle replacement after foot reconstruction. Jon had suffered without complaint through pain and discomfort that are unimaginable to most people. And Jon is one of the most genuinely kind and generous people I've ever known. If anyone could calm me down with a chat on Facebook, it would be Jon.

JON: Hi.

ME: Hey, Jon. How you doin'?

JON: How are you?

ME: We're good. Spending most of the summer here. I've got health problems that I hope we'll have answers about soon. Could be cancer. Just between you and me, okay?

JON: Have you heard the news?

ME: About what?

JON: Do you know about the Facebook lottery prize?

ME: [*pause*] Is this the Jon I know from Texas?

JON: All you have to do to check is go to [website URL deleted] and ask if your name is on the list of winners.

ME: Where did you and I work together, Jon?

JON: [*long pause*] I am a prof in Engelish [*sic*] at University of Central Texas. What is this?

ME: What's your dog's name?

JON: *Why are you asking all these questions?* All you have to do is go to the website to see whether you are winner. Its [*sic*] easy. Have you done that?

ME: Okay, Jon, go back up to the second message I sent you.

JON: Did you go to the website?

After I calmed down, I e-mailed Jon, whom I just realized I had imagined to be up at 4:00 a.m. in his time zone making new friends (that he already had) on Facebook. I warned him that his Facebook page had been hacked and that I had been in communication with the hacker but I hadn't talked about anything but my health.

Next day on Facebook I learned that dozens of Jon's friends had accepted his characteristically generous offer of a second friendship. There was much speculation about the personality characteristics of Fake Jon, whose account had already been deleted by Facebook central. Jon's daughter lamented that she felt she never really got to know her fake dad. Jon sent out a post explaining that technically his Facebook page had not been hacked in that no one's private information had been compromised; nothing not already available to the public had been taken from his page. He explained that the method of the imposter in this type of scheme includes copying all the public information (as well as photos) from a person's Facebook page and using that information to create an imposter page that is then used to attempt to swindle friends of the imposter's assumed identity.

The method is, thus, not technically hacking. It is termed instead . . . wait for it . . . *cloning*.

For the next several days I was burning with both shame and anger. In the wake of my initial feverous search for a self-diagnosis and of this cancerous cloning of Jon, the Internet seemed to me to be more and more ominously humanlike: capable (like your most well-meaning friends) of giving or confirming both good and bad advice and guilty (unlike your friends, if you choose them wisely) of the worst human impulses to deceive or take advantage for private gain.

Heather Responds to
"Don't Clone This"

Well, this is just how he is. Obsessed. He'll get an idea in his head, and then he's off to the Internet or off to the library or ordering this book or that online, burying himself in pdf printouts of articles— always looking, always searching. He's found typos in published statistical formulas this way, so he writes the authors and asks politely, "Did you mean to divide by whatsit rather than multiply?" And until he gets an answer, he's checking and rechecking, convinced that he's mistaken but still unable to get the formula to give him the result he wants. He wrote a program once that produced the results of four different statistical tests in a tabled row, yielding thousands and thousands of comparisons. As someone said in an online review of one of his books, "I see all the work that was put into this, but I have to ask *why?*"

So cancer is just the wrong thing for Don to get because he's going to be up all night for weeks looking for details that he is simply not going to be able to find, either because he's not trained as an oncologist and can't fully understand the articles he's reading or because there simply is no answer yet.

The Fake Jon episode is the kind of thing Don loves, eventually, when he gets over his initial rage. There's nothing at stake, it makes for a funny story in a mildly self-deprecating way, and it involves fraud that is ludicrously obvious, carried out by people probably dumb as bricks. This is why, Don says, he loves gangster movies: they are *all* about a bunch of people who think they know far more than they really do. He's watched *Goodfellas* so many times I simply cannot even be in the same room when he starts it. It drives me batty.

So blessings come in strange packages. If Fake Jon hadn't shown up, there is no telling how long Don would have been up that night. When he gets obsessive, he tends to binge—on information, on sugar, you name it, like the time we were moving from Texas to Illinois and my back went out. I was out of commission for about a month. Don did most of the packing, obsessively, until all hours of the morning, and to fuel these marathons he invited a monkey onto his back, fresh-baked bread (which I was making during the day) and syrup (low sugar, but still). One morning I woke up and I could hardly walk around the kitchen because there was something sticky everywhere on the floor. Don got up about noon and was acting all moody, so I didn't ask him about it. Later in the day I was looking for the loaf of bread I had just baked the day before.

"Do you know where the rest of the loaf of bread is?" I asked nervously.

"I stepped on it," Don said, matter-of-factly but cryptically.

"Excuse me?"

"I stepped on it."

"Oh."

It was one of those marital moments when you're dying to pursue a topic relentlessly but think better of it. A week later the full story came out.

"At 2:00 a.m. I realized I had to get that monkey off my back. I was eating more and more bread and more and more syrup and staying up later and later to pack, and I just lost it and threw the syrup container at the trash can and missed and it burst all over the kitchen floor [*other* mystery solved] and then I stomped on the bread and threw it away so I wouldn't find something else to put on it and eat it and stay up even later."

So if he's got a bee in his bonnet, when I tell Don not to stay up too late, I know I'm probably wasting my breath. But I tell him anyway.

Notes

1. *Understanding CLL/SLL (2016)*, 14,
2. "What Causes Lymphoma?"

Get the Fuck Out of My Way: I Have Cancer!

August 9

A FRIEND OF MINE FIRST suggested the title of this chapter as the slogan of a T-shirt to sell on a website devoted to this book if I published it. It's one of those funny, mood-lifting thought experiments she just throws out without effort because she's brilliant and hilarious. I prognosticate that sales of that T-shirt will trend virally when our demand for celebrities so far exceeds our supply that having cancer itself makes one a celebrity (even without being a famous athlete or actor). Or perhaps when cancer becomes culturally ironic, which in a celebrity culture may turn out to be inevitable, as is reflected in this quotation from CNN found on *Corpus of Contemporary American English:* "But Armstrong approached beating cancer with the same determination he brought to cycling."[1] Yes, if by *determination* one means *steroids.* See how easy it is?

If cancer ever becomes ironic, we will know then either (1) that there is a cure for all cancers, or (2) that we have lost our souls. The T-shirt will probably never sell in rock concert T-shirt numbers because no demographic, however goth, is ever going to be able to stand the look on strangers' faces when they discover that the T-shirt wearer actually has cancer. I mean, what would you say? And do people ever comment on others' T-shirts? Printed T-shirts seem to me to be like advertising or graffiti—too ubiquitous to bother with and of interest only to the wearer. Our T-shirt might be a bit different from most. It's shocking in three ways: the words *fuck* and *cancer* and the implicit promise of mortality. Hipsters, take note.

I've repurposed the T-shirt saying as a chapter title because it might increase sales of the T-shirt, the proceeds from which I promise to divide evenly between myself and my very talented friend. I don't know yet what my friend intends to do with her profits, but my share will go to the American Cancer Society. Cancer has already made me more generous, and more selfish too (see microscope shopping below). It has made me more generous because I suspect I have less time than I had thought to leave a lasting impression of generosity (I have a lot of lost ground to make up). And because I know that every single person now living will eventually realize—or already has, as I have—that the first thing that even the vaguest threat of serious illness rudely snatches from us is the illusion that we have all the time in the world. We never really had it in the first place.

In that spirit I am convinced that the T-shirt would serve as a thoughtful gift for a newly diagnosed cancer victim. It's a useful T-shirt because if that person is like me, he or she (or you) will be eager to get on with it—*it* being everything that can be done to diagnose, prognose, and get rid of the cancer now, right now! Nobody, whether at the blood lab or the bank or the grocery store, will dare cut in line in front of anyone wearing this T-shirt. This T-shirt says the wearer has cancer and is busy doing something about it.

So, like such an eager new cancer patient, I beat a hasty path to fetch my own personal copy of my blood lab work the very next morning, in spite of very short sleep. I forced myself not to look at the report until I had driven home because it was already hard enough to drive straight without calculating percentages for numbers of WBC (white blood cell counts), RBC (red blood cell counts), platelets, lymphocytes, and neutrophils, a few of the indicators that I had learned are important when one suspects leukemia.

Or at least this was the extent of my education gleaned from the Internet before my encounter with Fake Jon the night before. I also imagined the complete blood test and differential would have stamped in red letters CANCER or MONONUCLEOSIS or CAT SCRATCH FEVER across the front of it. I had forgotten the need for a lymph node biopsy, probably because I didn't understand why it was necessary in the first place. In any case I would have had a hard time keeping my truck in my own lane or even on the road. Plus I suspected that it would be bad luck to look at the report before I got home. It was like getting a letter from your preferred graduate school, a letter that would inform you of acceptance or *rejection*. Or a letter from the editor of a journal that you had submitted a scholarly paper to: acceptance or revision or *rejection*. I'd had lots of practice with this kind of magical thinking.

When I did get home and in a quiet place to read the blood report, I was surprised that nowhere on the blood report did the word *cancer* or *mononucleosis* or any of the other assorted wished-for ailments appear. Instead the flag *alert* appeared beside my count of 48,000 WBC per microliter. (You don't ever want to see that flag on your blood report. Just saying.) Even I could have supplied the word *alert,* both capitalized and italicized. But, but, but the pathologist noted, "Lymphocytes appear reactive." Within ten minutes I had discovered websites that taught me that reactive lymphocytes are sometimes indicative of infection. It took me days to discover that infections don't normally produce white blood cell counts in the 48,000 range and that leukemia cells can "appear reactive" as well. It was weeks before I realized that I didn't know what *reactive* even meant in "Lymphocytes appear reactive." I metaphorized *reactive* to mean "infectious" because I wanted an infection, not cancer. I think I also misunderstood the meaning because I was too busy looking up words I knew I didn't know, like *lymphocyte, neutrophil, blastoma,* and so on.

I could not understand why the blood report didn't provide a diagnosis since I had read in multiple places on the Web that all it took was a smear of blood on a slide to spot the distinctively engorged (the real meaning of *reactive* in the context of leukemia) and irregularly shaped nuclei of crowded leukemia cells. Besides, they all would look exactly the same, being clones. The images I had seen on the Web made spotting cancerous white blood cells seem as easy as spotting photoshopped celebrities in *Vanity Fair.* This stunning realization of the importance and ease of examining the shape of my white blood cells occurred to me just before I started shopping for medical-grade microscopes on the Internet. They are surprisingly cheap. For around $500 I could have overnight delivery of a 40x, 80x, 100x, 200x, 400x, 800x, 1,000x, or 2,000x digital microscope. I had spent more money on plane tickets to dozens of academic conferences that I didn't want to attend. Besides, who knows how many lab dollars this purchase could save?

Heather discouraged the purchase of the microscope, however reasonable, because I confessed that the next thing I would need, of course, was a flow cytometer, whose infinitely varied models appear to start in the range of $10,000. But you can get cheaper ones used. Flow cytometry, as I'll explain in confused detail later, appears to be necessary to determine the genetic modifications that one's cancer cells may have undergone. The pathology procedure is, supposedly, essential in even beginning to think about prognosis.

After a few days I convinced myself that when I met my oncologist during my first visit he would simply take another small blood sample, skip quietly next door to his laboratory, eyeball my lymphocytes, and perhaps shoot the whole works through his own flow cytometer. I had no clue at the time that it would be the surgeon, whom I had also yet to meet, who would extract the tissue specimen (a swollen lymph node) that would be used for both final diagnosis and flow cytometry results. Those results would not reach me for a full twenty days from the date of the initial blood test. I wouldn't first meet my oncologist for another seven days after that.

I'm as impatient to get to my vacation destination via an airplane as I am to get a cancer diagnosis and prognosis and treatment after visiting one or two labs, an oncologist, a surgeon, and a family physician. I find few things as exasperating as sitting in an airplane at 30,000 feet waiting for hours to touch down in some place utterly unlike the place I have just left, this new place implicitly promising me that I will, just by being there, discover new parts of myself that were inaccessible to me in the old place.

Why do I ever get on an airplane overstuffed with people, especially since the first thing I have to do is hand over all control for several hours? I do it because I normally sleep most hours of most flights. More frequently than not I'm asleep before the plane even takes off. When my sleep goes well I arrive refreshed and ready for action, and the best part is that I've skipped all that enforced patience, eating the "food," watching the movie, trying to read while crowded into a near-fetal position by other passengers and by the stingy anatomical design of the plane.

In the twenty days between the blood test and the return of the diagnosis and flow cytometry results after the lymph node biopsy, I did a lot of sleeping. I'm in talks with my T-shirt partner now about producing the shirts in extra long for double purposing as cancer patient jammies.

Heather Responds to
"Get the Fuck Out of My Way: I Have Cancer!"

Now you see what I meant in the last chapter. I wasn't exaggerating about his occasional obsessive behavior. He really did start shopping for medical-grade microscopes. I came home from work in the middle of this feverish frenzy. He couldn't wait for the diagnosis, so he was thinking about doing it himself with an expensive microscope. And that would be just like him. He's a gear head. To take just one of his many hobbies, he has eight guitars. Really?

Who needs eight guitars? How many guitars can you play at the same time? He used to have two motorcycles. He built one of them, and he's got all the tools he needed to do that, including an arc welder that trips the breaker box of the house practically every time he turns it on. He had a perfectly good motorcycle, which he donated to public radio, and they ended up selling it for $850, not a bad price for the buyer, given all the work and modifications that Don put into it. I asked him once, "Why didn't you just buy the motorcycle you wanted instead of taking apart this perfectly fine motorcycle and putting new everything on it: seat, shocks, handlebars, headlights, speedometer? I mean, speedometer? Did the second one measure the speed differently?" He told me that the journey is the destination. What?

One of our friends got it right. He asked Don, "Wouldn't it be safer to sell the motorcycle you built and keep the motorcycle you bought already assembled?" Don's answer: "I changed so many things on the old one that I might as well have built it." How are you even going to have a rational conversation with someone like that?

The "my white blood cells are reactive" phase was a classic example of confirmation bias: the tendency of humans to pay attention to what supports their hypotheses and to ignore that which would falsify their hypotheses. So now Don's already convinced he has an infection, not cancer. He finds that "reactive" white blood cells are indicative of infection and stops there—or rather, digs deeper into the evidence that infection causes reactive white blood cells, completely overlooking the facts that leukemia also causes reactive white blood cells and that he doesn't really know what *reactive* means when used to describe blood cells. Well, I get it. I prefer to stay in denial myself.

I think that the "reactive" white blood cells were Don's last lifeline to a cancer-free diagnosis, and I think he suspected that the lifeline was somehow based on flawed reasoning, because he was just beginning to realize how very complex oncology is.

Cancer research involves the study and treatment of a bundle of diseases with one or two common elements, but the peripheral symptoms, such as likelihood for metastasis, are as important to treatment and prognosis as the shared common elements.

Don did sleep a lot during this time, but I don't think it was solely escapism, as he implies here. I think he was exhausted from the constant thinking and research that he was trying to do. The doctors tell you to go home and live your life "normally." Impossible.

Notes

1. Davies, *The Corpus of Contemporary American English.*

Biopsy Surgery: Is Anything About This Going to Be Funny?

August 12

BEFORE I MET MY GENERAL SURGEON for the first time, I had read about all the pokey, cutty, ouchy procedures that might be required for a complete diagnosis, even though I was still hazy on why exactly a biopsy of a lymph node might be necessary when, again, I thought that all you'd have to do is look at my cloney white blood cells to find out whether I indeed had cancer. Later it became moderately clear to me that if you have small lymphocytic lymphoma, you also have some degree of chronic lymphocytic leukemia: if you find the former, you also find the latter. Besides, I was in no position to argue. I was holding out for a wicked sinus infection or at most mononucleosis, still hoping my medical team was wrong in suspecting cancer.

Among the procedures that I was prepared to demand fentanyl for were a lymph node biopsy, a bone marrow aspirate to look for the ultimate source of the problem (since leukemia begins in the bone marrow), and a spinal tap to see whether the cancer had metastasized to the spinal cord and the brain. These procedures are ranked roughly according to the degree that they inspired horror in me. All websites that I had consulted mentioned the possibility that any or all of these procedures could be done in a doctor's office with local anesthesia. Most also stated that some patients would find the procedures, particularly the bone marrow aspirate, uncomfortable, to say the least. The National Institutes of Health says that patients undergoing a bone marrow aspi-rate will experience a "painful sucking sensation as the marrow is removed" and that "if needed, [patients] are given medicine to help [them] relax."[1] I don't know whether this is merely gov-ernmental CYA language, but no one is giving me a painful suck-ing sensation without an argument. I believe in the miracles of modern medicine, but within that category I wholeheartedly endorse the miracles of modern anesthesia and sedation. I am not squeamish about surgery, but pain that is unnecessary is unnec-essary. Do what you want, but first dope me up or knock me out.

A man must have his principles, especially in this case, because according to Heather I have the lowest pain threshold that she's ever encountered in a human. What can I say? I'm sen-sitive. We make a bad pair in a medical situation in which I am asked to endure pain because she's a fainter. I could, if I were mean, make her faint simply by describing the details of one of my shoulder surgeries, which fascinate me. I've obsessively watched YouTube videos from beginning to end of arthroscopic repair of adhesive capsulitis, pausing at the really interesting bits, like the use of the wand that acts as a tiny meat grinder vacuum used to remove scar tissue in the frozen shoulder joint (which was the sole method used on my left shoulder). In the other procedure, used on my right shoulder, the wand is used to clean up some of the scar tissue, followed by a clipping and reattachment of the biceps tendon to the humerus to prevent the tendon from further cutting into the labrum. Now that's entertainment. Who could disagree?

I like to remind myself occasionally by viewing these videos how lucky I am to live in the age of arthroscopic surgery. I'm also filled with gratitude that I live in an age of effective and relatively safe general anesthesia, without which the surgery would be prac-tically impossible. Anesthesiology is so advanced that many sur-gical patients are given fentanyl even before general anesthesia.

Fentanyl, in case you don't know, is a strong opiate that nice anesthesiologists give their patients just prior to the patient being wheeled into the big bad operating room. (I have read just recently the alarming news that fentanyl has joined the group of opiates that some people are endangering their lives with. Sara Sidner reports for CNN that fentanyl "can be...50 times stronger than heroin.")[2] Medically administered fentanyl, according to my last operating room nurse, turns everyone into a comedian, although its medical purpose is to calm the anxious patient. When being wheeled through the doors into the operating room for my first shoulder surgery, about five minutes after a dose of fentanyl, I raised my arm as high as I could and yelled to everyone, "There's not a damned thing wrong with this shoulder." I still crack myself up with this one. My job as a properly medicated comedian is to give those poor overstressed nurses and doctors something to laugh at, you know, to release the tension in the room. I do my part. They do theirs.

The anesthesiologist for that first shoulder had almost certainly seen amateurs like me before though. Once I was settled on my gel bed and made all comfy with a blanket and oxygenated with a mask that smelled of strawberry gum, he held up an alarmingly large syringe with a milky white substance in it, explained that it was propofol, that it would put me to sleep in just a bit, right after I began to feel the cold creep up my arm, and oh, not to worry because even though the propofol would paralyze the muscles I use to breathe he would be "breathing for me." I was yelling, "What? How are *you* going to breathe for *me*?" and trying to lift the oxygen mask for him to hear me as I felt the distinct cold inch up my right arm. The next thing I knew I was in recovery.

I've had several surgeries requiring general anesthesia since that first shoulder arthroscopy. I always keep an eye out in the operating room for the anesthesiologist. Sometimes I see 'em; sometimes I don't. Heather and I have an ongoing argument about which of us is funnier. In the operating room the anesthesiologist always wins.

When I first met my laid-back general surgeon, who should

appear in a special GQ issue on cool and excellence, he explained that the only biopsy that my family physician had ordered was for the lymph node and that he, the surgeon, usually took them from the armpit—the axillary area. We decided together that he would take a node from the left axillary area because both left and right armpits were swollen with lymph nodes and because my right had been sliced open for the reattachment of my biceps tendon to my humerus. In truth, since it didn't matter, I wanted a new gnarly scar in my left armpit to match the one in my right—physical proof of my toughness beneath my catchy expletive-laden T-shirt. "So," he says, "if you are available Monday afternoon" (it just so happened I was), "my assistant will help set you up." I said, "So . . . will you be doing this here in your office?" He said, "Oh, no, in the hospital." This bit of news was an enormous relief to me because I couldn't imagine the amount of local anesthetic he would need to get me numb enough to lie still on the table, even with a load of fentanyl.

"I've only made that mistake once," he said with a small smile.

"What mistake?"

"Removing a lymph node in my office."

"Oh?"

"Yeah, it was a mess."

I didn't need to ask what kind of mess it must have been. The man is a surgeon, not an anesthesiologist. I'm certain the surgery was performed with excellent results; I doubt that anyone was laughing.

Heather and I had dinner last week with a friend and her visiting sister, a physician. I had fun talking with the doctor about surgeries and opiates. She told me about all her own surgeries and what opiates she herself tolerates well. Opiates have gotten me through the recovery periods of several surgeries. Given recent news of widespread opiate addition and overdosing in particular in the United States, some readers no doubt are uncomfortable with my praise of medically administered opiates prior to surgery and in recovery from surgery. In my "Afterward" I will return to this issue of opiate abuse, of which I am hyperaware, but for now, before any reader judges, first talk with anyone who has had shoulder surgery.[3]

Heather Responds to "Biopsy Surgery: Is Anything About This Going to Be Funny?"

I am the funny one. Let's just get that straight up front and then we can continue talking about the Center of the Universe Mr. Ha-Ha. Here's a hint about what's really going on here. Yes, Don has had a number of surgeries in recent years, probably above average for someone who has been relatively healthy. But all his examples of being "hilarious" are taken from times he was on pain medication. I have no doubt that he *thinks* he's funny, but that kind of misperception is just one of the reasons you are not allowed to drive under the influence of opiates. Your *judgment* is not to be trusted. And as he hints several times in this book, he's frequently not even sure about whether his oncology nurses are laughing with him or at him.

The same qualities that sometimes make him think he's the funniest person in the operating room are probably what make him generally a good patient. Nurses have told me that they like him, he's nice. He's always at least trying to have a good time, both when it's pretty easy to do because he's on fentanyl or when it's more of a challenge, like when he was getting six hours of chemotherapy in one day. I'll give him this much: he may not be the funniest one in the family, but he does try to be a good patient and he laughs at others' jokes as much or more than he laughs at his own. That's one reason why I know I'm the funny one in the house. I crack him up practically every day.

When he goes in for one of these surgeries, or even a colonoscopy, and he gets all medically induced funny, he comes home and tells and retells the "funny" stories endlessly. That's partly a result of the opiates as well. They affect your memory. He honestly can't remember that not five minutes previously he told me the same story.

That's how I knew the sidesplitting "There's not a damned thing wrong with this shoulder" story, and others you'll read in this book, would end up here.

To skip ahead a bit, Don still has a chemotherapy port in the right side of his chest, and they won't be giving him any fentanyl to remove it. We'll see how funny he is after he comes home from having that procedure done with not much more than a subdermal local anesthetic like lidocaine, which burns like fire when it goes in.

And yeah, I've always been a fainter, but it turns out I'm not the only fainter in the family.

Notes

1. Gersten, "Bone Marrow Aspiration."
2. Sidner, "Fentanyl."
3. "Living Through Rotator Cuff Injury and Surgery."

Waking Up

August 15

O UT OF ALL THE NURSES who have helped me, some of my favorites have been recovery nurses, whether for relatively minor procedures like a colonoscopy or more complex procedures like shoulder surgery. They are almost always really nice people who help wake you up gently. Where else does that ever happen? They help orient you to the world of consciousness again, because at least in my experience propofol takes a person to the land of no memory, where you might even forget you're a patient.

On first reaching groggy consciousness, my first thoughts are usually "Why does my [*insert name of body part here*] hurt as if someone has set it on fire and then tried to put out the fire by stomping on it?" followed by the far more clichéd "Where am I?" These two questions usually occur at almost the same moment, thus disproving the local assumption, popular in my house among cats, dog, and human, that I cannot think of more than one thing at a time. After another surgery, this time to clean out an infection in my left axillary area, resulting from who-knows-what some two weeks after the lymph node biopsy, I woke up slurring my words (normal under the circumstances) and repeatedly asking the question "What seems to be the problem here?" with no particular problem in mind (distinctively abnormal). I don't think I was using my indoor or recovery room voice either because the nurse reassured me that "everything is okay" and requested politely,

"Please speak quietly. I think you are disturbing other patients!" I don't know why I woke up with such an imperious attitude except that perhaps I considered myself an expert on surgery by that point and thought I was the chief surgeon on a well-written medical TV drama. Another reason I like recovery room nurses is that they sometimes, depending on the surgery, give me a small whiskey shot of liquid morphine. That nearly always does two things: almost immediately it makes me completely forget my questions and gets me going as if I was born to be the most garrulous and grateful cowboy in the dustiest bar in the West.

By the time recovery nurses decide that the pain is under control, that I can hold my morphine, and that I can be trusted to live another day without dying of any of the various ailments they track with sober eye—hypothermia, low blood pressure, poor oxygen absorption, weak pulse (all of which can be brought on by extended unconsciousness induced by propofol)[1]—I usually know (1) where they attended university, (2) their major (my last was a double major in history and English before she went to nursing school), (3) whether they have pets and what their names are, and (4) how they react to flattery, the last because I usually develop mild crushes on recovery nurses, male or female, young or old or in between.

It's the morphine, of course, mixed with the joy of being alive, topped off by my being for a good period of time the sole and intense center of attention for another human being. The last is the secret, of course, to getting anyone to fall in love with you if they are at all predisposed to do so. There is the occasional nurse who is far above my league of bullshit, and we both know it. I'm sure that all recovery nurses promptly forget about me upon the arrival of the next groggy soul in pain, but for me the attachment lingers for the rest of the day, like the bittersweet mood you get when you've finished a book that was so good you're sorry to leave that world. Recovery rooms are magical; I normally look around squinty-eyed at the other patients and try to radiate my love for life and everything in it, at least on a good day. People who know me know this isn't normal. But nothing about surgery is.

My only negative experience in a recovery room wasn't really the recovery nurse's fault; it was a communication problem. My first orthopedist wanted to cure my adhesive capsulitis in my shoulder without surgery but rather with medieval methods such as hanging my entire body weight from my hands, thus stretching my arms straight above my head until I could stand it no more and dropped to the ground in agony. There were two months of painful physical therapy as well, none of it fruitful. I changed surgeons. The new one took a good look at the X-rays and MRI and pronounced me incurable by medieval torture and promptly scheduled me for arthroscopic surgery. When the anesthesiologist determined through examination of records that I had been prescribed oxycodone for my physical therapy, he decided not to use an anesthetic shoulder block after the surgery, which is common protocol because immediate post-operative pain is potentially very high for shoulder surgery. Under normal conditions the anesthetic shoulder block would have been good for several hours and would have made supplemental pain killers unnecessary until it wore off. My anesthesiologist quite appropriately did not want to take the risk of sending me home with a shoulder block and having it wear off early because of an increased tolerance to pain medication. His decision was for the recovery nurse to first treat with morphine and then send me home with another prescription for oxycodone. The problem was that no one had told the recovery nurse that the normal protocol had been changed for my surgery.

When I woke up in recovery, a grotesque comedy of errors ensued in which I felt as if I was having my arm amputated at the shoulder by an angry bear; the recovery nurse insisted that I should not be experiencing so much pain with a shoulder block. I unsuccessfully tried to summarize the complicated plot. The recovery nurse knocked me out again with something (he never told me what) in my IV while he got the story straight from the surgeon and anesthesiologist, after which I was given morphine. I was then wheeled to another room for further "observation," not "recovery," where I met my first truly unpleasant nurse, who insisted that I must "own" my pain, and that if I didn't own my pain and tell her on the record that I was safe to go home with that level of pain, she was going to check me in overnight and "neither of us want *that,* do we?" The problem was that it took a while for the morphine to take the ragged, screeching edge off the pain in my shoulder. Once the morphine kicked in, I said I was ready to own my pain and go home. I think the nurse and I were equally glad to be rid of each other. I was angry for two days after that experience. I felt disrespected and humiliated.

Humiliation in hospitals is a rare emotion in my experience. Almost everyone I meet is kind, and in surgery you pretty much elect to give up privacy when you hand your body over, clad in nothing but a flimsy gown that doesn't even close properly in the back, to what is essentially a small group of strangers. Although I don't actively worry about it, I've had enough surgeries under general anesthesia to wonder about, oh, let's say, a certain male body part waking up early and rather vigorously to take a look around, perhaps to see what all the fuss is about and to say, "Hey, I'm here." The Internet tells me that erections do occur while patients are under anesthesia, but as I said, I'm not worried about it. I voluntarily give up the right to erectile privacy when I agree to surgery with general anesthesia.

Aside from hilarious and uplifting animal videos, the Internet, or at least *my* Internet, can be a dark place, full of dire pronouncements about the likely outcomes of this or that cancer diagnosis or therapy. Because the Internet is full of concerns that are characteristically human—sex, mortality, Facebook friends (Real Jon or Fake Jon)—it can occasionally cast just the right ludicrous light on my obsessional googling. In my overly diligent Internet research, I learned that a disorder termed *priapism* does rarely occur under the influence of propofol. The name itself of this dangerous and painful disorder (a "prolonged" and "usually painful" erection) is, uh, perhaps flattering in a backhanded way for most males.[2] It is also the only example of humor that I am aware of in what seems to me to be the normally somber obscurantist world of medical terminology (priapism comes from Priapus: "A Graeco-Roman god of procreation and fertility, usually represented as a small, deformed figure with an enormous phallus").[3]

Expecting chemotherapy, should I enter that chapter of the experience, to be considerably less amusing than surgery, I offered my current surgeon the opportunity to go back in and remove all my estimated five-hundred-plus lymph nodes and leave just the spleen. He politely declined.

One last curiosity: leukemia is also a risk factor for priapism, with or without propofol.[4]

Heather Responds to
"Waking Up"

You see what I'm talking about here, right? If he had known the term priapism before his surgeries, which I can almost guarantee you he did not (I'm the Scrabble champ in the house too), he would have used it in some lame joke in the operating room, and everyone would have said, "Ha ha, that's funny" (and to the anesthesiologist: "How soon can you knock out Woody Allen here?"). And then I would have heard about how funny he was and how funny everybody thought he was and so on. And can I just ask whether anyone is really surprised that Don's example of humor in his Google-obsessed world is a dick joke?

What he didn't go on and on about here (and I'm surprised he didn't because he normally doesn't fail to elaborate on stories about pain) is that he spent two solid months in physical therapy and doing torturous exercises at home every single day under the direction of his first orthopedist to try to loosen up the adhesions in his shoulder. If a doctor tells Don that he ought to be able to do something, well, he's going to do it, especially if it involves will-power. He would hang from the opening to the attic four or five times a night, each time yelling in pain, and then when he let go and the adhesions snapped his shoulder back into the inflamed joint he would double over with the ache and groan some more. Then there were the endless stretches meant to break up the adhesions in the shoulder. He would lie on his side with his arm bent at the elbow but the lower part of the arm perpendicular to his body, before taking the other arm and pushing backward. If you try it—and you shouldn't—you will probably experience some pain. Most people's shoulders aren't meant to bend in that direction much. Don's wouldn't bend in that direction at all. He would watch TV and push and push and push and yell and cuss about it each time. If he had taken a pain pill to keep the pain under control, he would work even harder, sometimes an hour or two at a time, watching some program. The shoulder just would not give. It was like watching Sisyphus, only in this case Sisyphus couldn't even budge that rock. Don never made any progress at all.

One reason Don worked so hard to try to break up the adhesions from that first frozen shoulder was that he was trying to avoid the type of surgery that the first orthopedist had planned, which was to knock Don out, probably with propofol, and get two or three strong-armed nurses to help him break up the adhesions by force. Don had of course done the Internet research and discovered that many people's shoulders became worse after such manipulation by brute force. The pain certainly gets worse as well, at least for most people for a while. Don's physical therapists finally told him the same thing when it was clear that Don and they weren't going to be able to move the shoulder by normal physical therapy manipulation.

I have to admit that during physical therapy and those exercises at home Don hardly joked about it at all. He didn't think anything about it was funny. And, even though I'm the funny one, I wasn't laughing either.

Notes

1. "Propofol Side Effects."
2. Senthilkumaran et al., "Propofol and Priapism"; "Priapism: Overview."
3. *Oxford English Dictionary.*
4. "Priapism: Symptoms and Causes."

How to Talk to People About Your Cancer

August 19

MY GENERAL SURGEON told Heather after the biopsy surgery, while I was in recovery, that he had to remove three lymph nodes rather than one because they were matted and impossible to separate. Good: the pathologist has plenty of tissue to work with. Bad: it was an indication that my lymph nodes were so swollen with white blood cells that the lymph nodes themselves were crowding one another, much as the white blood cells were crowding not only one another but also other, functioning cells like red blood cells and platelets. Fatigue is sometimes an early indication of CLL/SLL, even before the disease starts to crowd out oxygen-bearing red blood cells, because it takes energy to make all those useless cloned white blood cells. The combination of that fatigue with the psychological sucker punch of a tentative cancer diagnosis makes for a lethargic funk that is hard to break out of. So how do you combat that? You *do* something, dammit! My eternal urge to fix things applied squarely to myself. But the reality is "Okay, everybody, let's wait for an official diagnosis!" Next best thing: talk to people in the waiting room we all share.

After my family physician made the tentative diagnosis of cancer, Heather and I talked about who we should tell. At the beginning the diagnosis seemed like news that could be controlled if we were just careful about it. I've never had to decide when to tell everybody that "we" were pregnant, but those of you who have know how tricky all medical announcements, even good ones, can be.

I knew that telling my mom and stepmom would be upsetting because my dad had just died in February, five months earlier. Mom went straight to the core logical problem: "You're not supposed to die before me. I'm your mother!" Both moms had good advice: get plenty of rest, eat more, and try not to worry, all of which practical advice is better than searching the Internet at 3:00 a.m. We also told a handful of close friends. We decided not to tell anyone else unless the lymph node biopsy confirmed a diagnosis of cancer. Cancer gifts are probably more awkward to return than even wedding gifts for a cancelled wedding. "Oh, sorry, I was sure I was dying of cancer but it turns out that it's just mononucleosis. Thanks for your thoughtful card and your prayers of support and the Navajo bear 'strength' fetish. Should I just keep that?" No less awkward: I'd have to return my cancer T-shirt or simply stuff it away in the bottom of a drawer to be forgotten.

The surgeon made it clear that the final diagnosis would be made by the pathologist who reviewed my lymph node biopsies. I didn't know how the diagnosis would be reported to me, so I stayed close to the home telephone, whose number we had given all physicians involved so far. This was my first mistake. My home telephone is the equivalent of a junk e-mail folder. Eighty percent of calls are politicians and supporters of politicians, the remainder usually wrong numbers or scam artists. Most people who know us, including our vets, call us on our cell phones.

The surgeon called with the diagnosis two days after the biopsy surgery, I think toward 5:00 p.m., but I'm not sure. Naturally, I had even studied up on how cancer patients receive and react to diagnoses of cancer. It seems that reactions to leukemia diagnoses are quite varied, ranging from shock to calm acceptance.[1] My own romantic cinematographic reaction, I thought, would be the sensation of everything being projected in slow motion: later I would remember seeing a dove alight uncertainly on a branch outside my window, see my cat, Lyndon, notice that dove as he sat on the windowsill, watch the dust motes visible in a beam of late-afternoon sunshine on my first-floor home office. Truth is, I don't remember any of that—so much for my choreographed transcendent reaction—but I do remember I picked up without even checking the caller ID.

"Hello?"

"Mr. Hardy?"

"Yes?"

"This is your surgeon, Dr. ——."

"Yes?"

"The pathology report is back from your lymph node biopsy."

"Yes?"

"You have chronic lymphocytic leukemia and small lymphocytic lymphoma."

"Oh."

"Your family physician has told you that this is usually highly treatable?"

"Yes."

"Do you have any questions for me?"

"Uh, no, I don't think so, thanks."

"Okay. I will see you for your appointment to check on the stitches. Are you having any problem with the incision or the drain?"

"No, Doctor, thank you for calling."

"I'll see you in a week."

"Okay, good-bye."

"Good-bye."

I can't say for sure whether the doctor was as laconic as I represent him here, but it is his nature to be soft spoken. I don't remember anything other than that the surgeon told me that I had CLL/SLL, that he asked about the incision and Jackson-Pratt (JP) Drain, and that I was so emotionally numb that I wanted to just hang up on him but didn't, partly because he himself sounded so sad about the diagnosis that I wanted to apologize for having cancer.

The incision, the lymph node extractions, and the JP Drain were still causing me pain in spite of the oxycodone I was prescribed (I wasn't allowed to drive until after the four days I was to take the oxy). The incision, about 3.5 inches long, was heavily bandaged, and extruding from one end of that bandage was the drip line to my JP Drain, what they called a grenade in the recovery room. The grenade is a collapsible bulb that suctions blood, stray tissue, and lymph fluid through its line until the lymph vessels exposed by the biopsy shrink and heal. Once the collected fluid fell below 30 milliliters per twenty-four-hour-period, I was told, I could come in and have a nurse remove the grenade and the drip line. Over a period of about a week, the liquid turned from red (mostly blood) to yellow (mostly lymph fluid), mixed with bits of tissue, some up to an inch long. Absolutely fascinating to me—no doubt grotesque to others.

But my telephone conversation with my surgeon wasn't the most emotional conversation I had that week. Just the day before, the day after the surgery, I had had a rather unfriendly chat with a "police officer."

"Hello?"

"Mr. Hardy?"

"Yes?"

"Mr. Hardy, I'm calling from the police department about a bench warrant for your failure to appear in court."

"Excuse me?"

"Mr. Hardy, you have a bench warrant for your arrest for failure to appear. You can either turn yourself in to the main headquarters of the police department today or you can take care of this with a $1,000 fine, payable with a credit card."

"What? I don't understand what you are talking about. This is impossible."

"Mr. Hardy, it is not impossible. You failed to appear in court on July 29 and thus have a bench warrant for your arrest. Do you wish to take care of this over the telephone?"

"Okay, what is your name?"

"Officer John ——."

"Okay, Officer ——, what is your supervisor's name?"

"My supervisor?"

"Yes, your immediate superior officer."

"Buford ——."

"*Buford?!* You have got to be kidding me! Look, John, I've just been diagnosed with cancer, and if I knew who you really were and where you were right now, I would fuck you up."

"Mr. Hardy, you sound impaired. How about I send a police unit over to your home right now to search it for contraband?"

"Bring it on, asshole!"

Officer —— hung up. I didn't even have a chance to say goodbye. Of course, I exercised all reasonable care and discovered through Internet research, mere child's play at this point, that a bench warrant telephone scam had been reported in our area recently.

I guess all I'm trying to say here is that you have to share when you're ready. Talk to your family because they are there for you just as you are there for them; don't feel that you have to apologize to your doctors for being sick; and screen all calls.

Heather Responds to
"How to Talk to People About Your Cancer"

I remember clearly when Don called my office and reported that his surgeon had just called him with the pathology report. I came home right away, and we talked about what would be happening soon, including a call from an oncologist, whom Don would see to talk about treatment options. Don had read about the "watch and wait" procedure with CLL/SLL, but we didn't know yet how advanced or aggressive his cancer was. It didn't seem *that* aggressive to either of us. Don had lost a lot of weight, but that had happened so long ago we weren't really thinking of that as one of the symptoms. He had swollen lymph nodes and elevated white blood cell counts, but the lymph nodes didn't seem horribly swollen, and Don's Internet research told him that the white blood cell count in stable CLL/SLL patients could go a lot higher than what he was walking around with at that time. He had staged his cancer as probably a 2 on the 4-point scale. What I didn't tell him is that I had gone on the MD Anderson site and using their criteria it was at least a 3. Don isn't the only one who knows how to google his way to bad news. (Remember, I once convinced myself through Internet searches that I had rabies.) I decided to wait and let his doctor tell him.

Oddly, what Don doesn't tell me about right away are things like the conversation he had with the fake Officer John. Don is very strange that way. He has a fascinating telephone conversation with a scam artist, spots him, and calls him out, and he doesn't tell me until three days later. He just casually mentions it at dinner later that week. Perhaps if it had happened in the OR while he was drugged with fentanyl, I would have heard about it sooner—and more often.

"Oh, somebody pretending to be from the local police station called and said that I had a bench arrest warrant out for me."

"You have a what?!"

"A bench warrant. I'm not even sure I know what that is. But the phone call is bullshit."

"I know what a bench warrant is. It's an arrest warrant usually issued by a judge when you don't show up for court."

"Well, like I said, it's bullshit."

"Why didn't you tell me?"

"I didn't think it was important."

"Not important that the police have a warrant for your arrest?"

"But they don't, or they didn't. It was a scam. The guy said his supervising officer's name was Buford, for Christ's sake."

"You need to tell me about these things a little closer to the event. What if it had been real?"

"But it wasn't."

And so on. Don hates telephones, maybe because he's always home to catch the wacko calls in the middle of the day. It's gotten so that he usually doesn't answer the landline at all. And he's also horrible about his cell phone. He claims not to know what text messaging is. He knows what it is. He just doesn't want to do it.

Notes

1. "Leukaemia: Reactions to the Diagnosis."

Keeping My Story Straight

August 21

AS SOON AS I RECEIVED the diagnosis of CLL/SLL, I started making big ambitious plans for the coming semesters, even though I'd yet to talk to an oncologist. Obviously I would be going into chemotherapy. Obviously I would be taking leave from teaching and service to lessen the serious threat of communicable infection of any sort, infection that chemotherapy makes increasingly likely the more people one interacts with. I would continue to do my research alone at home, which is how I do most of that part of my job anyway. I had firm plans to be in remission by January and come back full-time to work with buckets of energy for teaching, service, and research, and I would be ready to go skiing in the spring. For the ski slopes I would obviously need a T-shirt that declared my recent victory over cancer. I thought about the "I'm Making Cancer My Bitch!" T-shirt but was bothered by the implied long-term commitment to the relationship. There was also the implicit threat that the relationship might be reversed. After much deliberation I decided on the "Hey, Cancer, You Picked the Wrong Bitch!" T-shirt, which I was surprised and happy to discover comes in a men's size and cut. There is a "Hey, Cancer, You Picked the Wrong Chump!" T-shirt, but that seems like your dad's or even granddad's T-shirt, not the T-shirt for a hip survivor of cancer on the ski runs in the sunny days of April, when all the cool kids are wearing swimsuits on the slopes.[1]

I had read on the Web the laundry list of side effects from the chemotherapy for CLL/SLL (nausea, fatigue, weight loss, loss of appetite, mouth sores, hair loss),[2] but what pharmaceuticals couldn't take care of, I was going to beat with a positive attitude and sweet mother nature: plenty of rest and green and herbal teas. I don't have that much hair left to lose anyway. The chemotherapy cocktail would probably be fludarabine, cyclophosphamide, and rituximab (with the completely uninspiring acronym of FCR).[3] It sounds more like a personnel document that everyone forgets to fill out on time every year than a combination of drugs designed to beat leukemia/lymphoma into a whimpering submissive disease, still probably hiding out in the bones somewhere, but at least afraid to show its humiliated face for a few years.

That was my story—and my plan—at least until I met my oncologist for the first time. He gently and persuasively explained at length that in spite of what clearly appeared to me to be an alarming rise in the number of white blood cells circulating in my body and in spite of enlarged lymph nodes that were close enough to the surface of the skin to be visible, we would do best in my case to be cautious and enter a watch and wait mode, primarily because there are no experimental data to show that early treatment is superior in survival statistics to watching and waiting, waiting specifically until symptoms become numerous and serious enough to start negatively affecting quality of life. So I will see my oncologist once a month to monitor white blood cell count as well as other important indicators such as red blood cells and platelets, and to watch for other symptoms should they arise.

Among the things that I have to do now that I didn't do before the diagnosis, although I've probably had CLL/SLL for at least two years, are

- avoid raw fish;
- avoid raw vegetables, including salads, at restaurants;
- wash my vegetables and fruit compulsively, like a raccoon;

- make and keep all recommended physician appointments;
- google every single word a physician uses in my presence.

And among the signs that it is time to break out the not-so-fun chemicals are two episodes of night sweats within one week, a temperature of over 100.5 degrees lasting for a week, doubling or tripling of size of visible lymph nodes, enlargement of liver and/or spleen, low red blood cell counts and/or platelet counts, and 10 percent unexplained weight loss in six months. Some websites suggest that hitting a temperature of 100.5 alone is reason enough to call your oncologist.[4] This is a lot to explain to folks who haven't recently talked to an oncologist, a surgeon, and a family physician about CLL/SLL and haven't spent two months reading everything they could excavate about the disease from the Internet.

Rather wisely, I think now, although in truth it was probably accidental, I had not told anyone but family about my surely triumphant chemotherapy and recovery plans for fall and spring, so all I had to do after my first visit with my oncologist—the visit that dismantled *my* elaborate plans—was tell family that my oncologist had decided to put me in the watch and wait category and see me every month for regular and close monitoring. My mom, who was once a nurse, said, "That doesn't sound much like treatment to me. Are you comfortable with your doctor?" I said, "Well, the way I understand it is that the treatment is only a hair better than the disease and that it's better to wait until the disease is actively trying to kill me before we go after it with toxic drugs." I invented this completely bogus medical weighting of risk/benefit myself because even though I know it's a grotesque caricature of the truth, it's easy for me to remember so that I can keep my story straight.

Heather is the dean of the College of Liberal Arts at the University of Nevada, Reno, where I work. One of the things this means is that many more people on campus vaguely know *about* me (that I exist) than actually know me. Even though my condition wasn't generally known, in a meeting of administrators of the university, one turned to Heather and asked in a hushed voice, "How's Don?" You guessed it: I've never met this person so concerned with my welfare, or perhaps really only concerned with how Heather is holding up. It was a kind thing to ask, I think. Heather said, "Oh, thank you for asking. What have you heard?" demonstrating just how diplomatic she can be in slightly awkward situations. The kind-hearted individual replied, "I've heard that he has cancer and is steadfastly refusing all treatment." Heather quietly corrected the misunderstanding, and the larger meeting proceeded without further discussion of oncology, so far as I know.

Just because I myself have a story that is relatively straight most of the time doesn't mean that there aren't alternative versions of myself out there bumping up against the self that I've created through the story I tell, sort of like a collision of two of the many parallel universes that some physicists theorize exist. If we live within a multiverse (with infinite universes) rather than within a single universe, there exists somewhere, far away, at least one Don Hardy who has CLL/SLL and is making exactly the same decisions that I am making under the same circumstances. Also perhaps just as far away or even farther, there is logically at least one Don Hardy who has CLL/SLL and is like me in every other detail except that he is refusing treatment for cancer as if he's planning to go Chuck Norris on it all by himself and thus send the cancer into remission by unrelenting steely-eyed intimidation combined with superior martial arts skills. I sincerely wish that Don Hardy all the luck in his world.[5] And I wonder what the Heather in that universe would have replied to the question of how that Don was doing.

Heather Responds to
"Keeping My Story Straight"

I find it somewhat ironic that Don titled this chapter the way he did, because he is *the* most inconsistent, changeable person I know. It might better have been titled "Keeping My Current Story

Straight." It's not that he's a liar. He can't lie successfully, I think, because he thinks everything he says is funny and that it's a good joke to lie. So since he has no poker face either, all I have to do is watch his expression. There's a look he gets: a corner of his lips curls ever so slightly and the eyes get all expectant, as if they're saying, "I'm lying to you. See, it's a game. Now you try to tell whether I'm lying." See how stupid this is? He's like our dog when he's desperately running through all the tricks he knows, unbidden, hoping to get a treat as a reward. Since Don's not really trying to fool anyone (unlike Lyle the dog), the right corner of his mouth turns up. He's got a tell, but he doesn't believe it. This is the same guy who thinks he could be a mobster or a university administrator. Within a year he'd be under the cement foundation of a new student success center on campus.

One of the stories he cannot keep straight for more than a month at a time, normally, is what he likes to eat. This inconsistency goes beyond what I call his food enthusiasms: nuts, which he was on for six months; peanut butter and jelly sandwiches, which he currently has for breakfast every single morning; and sorbet or frozen yogurt for dessert every night. He embraces these enthusiasms wholeheartedly until—suddenly—he's off them.

He's erratic about television preferences as well. He's gotten several seasons into television programs and suddenly declared one evening, "I don't like this program anymore": *The Walking Dead, Downton Abbey, Under the Dome.* So there we are, right in the middle of zombie slaughter (it's pretty much the same from episode to episode) and he decides he's tired of zombie slaughter. I'm inventing motivation here for him because he never articulates his reasons, except that once he muttered something about *Downton Abbey* being like a soap opera, which is similar to discovering one day that *The Walking Dead* is about zombie slaughter. On the other hand, he's watched all of *The Sopranos, The Shield,* and *The Wire* more than once each. And I've already told you about *Goodfellas.* The same is true of all three *Godfather* movies. If I have to watch any of them again, I'll scream. You see the pattern. I think he really does fantasize about being a mobster. But mobsters have to be able to lie with a straight face.

The account about the fellow administrator who had heard that Don was refusing all treatment is true. He heard that story via a circuitous route typical of a smallish city like Reno. It taught both me and Don something: you can't control your story in the public arena. We had talked, probably with more than one friend, about whether we ought to announce yet again to family and friends what was going on with treatment or what the watch and wait plan was. Most likely "watch and wait" got turned into "he's refusing treatment." What are you going to do about that? Stories beget stories.

And if one story begets another, you can't keep your story straight. If I can't figure out what he's going to want to eat on a given day, we can't expect people who don't even know him to keep the cancer treatment story straight, especially when it seems so counterintuitive: "You have cancer, so what we're going to do is watch and wait until it gets bad." Wait until cancer gets bad? "And by the way, go and try to live your life normally." Of all the possible universes out there, this "live normally" advice has to be easier in some than others. But really, the advice to stay in the now is probably good wherever you find yourself.

Notes

1. For cancer T-shirts, see ChucklenutShirts.com.
2. "Chemotherapy for Chronic Lymphocytic Leukemia."
3. "FCR Chemotherapy."
4. "Fevers: When Cancer Becomes an Emergency."
5. *The Fabric of the Cosmos;* Vilenkin and Tegmark, "The Case for Parallel Universes"; Hooper, "Multiverse Me"; Kriss, "The Multiverse Idea Is Rotting Culture"; Folger, "Science's Alternative to an Intelligent Creator."

I'd Rather Not Know Anyway

August 26

IN MY LAST APPOINTMENT with my favorite psychologist, about five years ago, I asked whether I should come back for a checkup every once in a while. He replied, "You are certainly welcome. I'd be happy to see you. But you already know what I would tell you."

Two years earlier I had walked into that same psychologist's office, sat down on his couch, and for an hour proceeded to rock and gibber to myself like a cheap wind-up doll in an effort to push panic (about everything that my sticky mind could grab hold of) out of the bottom of my feet and through the floor and into the ground. Two years later his implicit denial of my suggestion that there were still yet-unplumbed depths of my mind was one of the most liberating things a doctor has ever said to me. The science of psychology to this point has done all it can for me. I'm not cured, but I walk the earth with the anti-venom always on my person. That is, among many, many other hard-won admissions and insights: "What other people think of me is none of my business." I would have never guessed during that first visit that any doctor was capable of (1) understanding why my mind was so grabby and sticky, and (2) teaching me how to Teflon-coat it so that even the most obsessive and irrational of fears and self-hatreds and even needs to know would slide off the surface without a trace.

In 1962, when I was six years old, I had a very bad sore throat. Before I knew it my mom and I were walking through the front doors of Denton Regional Hospital. I was hungry, because when the sore throat got bad enough that it brought on fever and a head-ache, my mom recognized the symptoms as indicative of tonsilli-tis and got me to the hospital fast before I'd had dinner. It was now 7:00 p.m., and I was hungry. I asked when we would get something to eat, and she said, "You probably won't eat until after the sur-gery." Being the child of a nurse who worked in a hospital, I knew that surgery was serious business, and I was so fearful I nearly bolted right there and then. My last question, which I would not have dared ask out loud, was, "Will I get to say good-bye to Laddie [our collie]?" I don't blame my mom; I look back now and know that I couldn't have done a better job myself as a parent. She had somehow gotten me to the hospital without my even suspecting what was coming, and that included at least a forty-minute drive from our house on a farm into Denton, which I viewed then as the big city.

The only person I was angry with about my tonsillectomy for a number of years was, you guessed it, the anesthesiologist, who I later learned used ether, which has a dense, foul yet slightly sweet petroleum odor, as I remember it. The anesthesiologist poured what looked to me like a haphazard unmeasured amount of ether on the mask I wore. I immediately tried to squirm away. The doc-tors and nurses had, of course, anticipated this reaction, so one of the terrifying feelings was that I couldn't escape their tight grip on me. The anesthesiologist said, "It smells bad, doesn't it?" I groaned. "If you don't like it, you can puff it away." This encouraged me to take one or two deep breaths to blow it away, making the smell even that much more horrible, and the next thing I remember I was waking up in recovery with a disappointingly small amount of ice cream waiting in a cardboard cup with what looked like a toy wooden spoon affixed to the top.

So some withholding of information is a gift. I will forever be grateful to our friend who contracted mononucleosis just about the same time I was diagnosed with CLL/SLL. She had probably been infected with the virus during a party at her house for her daughter's thirty best teenage friends. She and I had lunch the day before she became symptomatic with mononucleosis, at which lunch she shared with me half her sandwich. On the day that would mark the six-week incubation period of mononucleosis for me, she told me that she had heard from Heather of my increasing anxiety about preferring mononucleosis to CLL/SLL. She had gritted her teeth and carried the anxiety for all those days, not wanting to worry me with the possibility of coming down with an infectious disease directly on top of being diagnosed with cancer. Heather knew the entire mononucleosis story from our mutual friend and uttered not a word about it until I was safely past the incubation period. In medicine, family, friendship, and marriage, there are sometimes angels who shoulder our suffering by hiding both truth and ignorance from us, out of duty and love, while also sharing the occasional sandwich.

Heather Responds to
"I'd Rather Not Know Anyway"

Apart from the shoulder surgeries, the biopsies, the cancer itself, even the depression, the most frightening illness I've seen Don go through were the two years of anxiety disorder. So it is good that he may very well now be walking around in blissful self-congratulatory ignorance of some things, but really, who isn't? There are days I can't listen to NPR. There's sometimes just too much bad news out there: the wars, the shootings, the tsunamis, the earthquakes, the climate, the cost of healthcare, the economy, politics. I personally think that we are here on earth to learn. Learning is different from knowing.

It is true that Don is frequently overly concerned with what others think of him. Hence his psychotherapist's advice that what other people think, even about Don, is none of his business. I think that honestly came as both a revelation and a relief to Don. In an earlier chapter, I hinted at another frequent pronouncement to Don from his psychotherapist: "You're wrong." The severe anxiety that Don went through for a couple of years manifested primarily as completely false ideation (resulting in deeply embedded false recollections)—that he had run over a child, that he had plagiarized both of his books, that he had thrown important notes of mine away. These are just a few examples of the alarming products of his uncontrolled apocalyptic imagination. So he spent two years learning that he was wrong about almost everything that had preoccupied his chronically panicked mind.

I think for both of us as we go through his chemotherapy and live with the possibilities and limitations of future treatment, our challenge is to realize that all we can do is the best we can throughout the process without expecting to know much of anything about the future with certainty. Those years of living with Don's insistent but constantly wrong mind have prepared us well for a long period of uncertainty.

So the title of Don's chapter "I'd Rather Not Know Anyway" is paradoxical because in a sense he already has his wish fulfilled.

Quit That Looking at Me!

September 2

THE FIRST SUPERPOWER I'd wish for is the ability to cure cancer with something positive, like a good belly laugh, which would substantially increase the income of good stand-up comics and comedy writers and weed out the bad ones. But since the cure for cancer may be further away than a cloak of invisibility, I'll take the cloak of invisibility as second choice. I think many cancer patients would, or at least I would, be eager to sign up for a phase 1 clinical trial for a cloak of invisibility. Perhaps—really, no doubt in many ways—I am spoiled.

I probably need something a bit more mundane than a cloak of true invisibility—perhaps just a cloak that would shield cancer patients from all the various indignities of the body and mind that cancer seems to show up with uninvited. "Hey, I'm here, and I've brought all my least presentable but closest friends with me. Hope you don't mind. Make room, please." I've been spared thus far all of the more extreme tortures of cancer. And I haven't yet entered chemotherapy, which the more I read about the more I fear, maybe more than the cancer itself.

A friend's husband recently went through chemotherapy for testicular cancer. In the middle of his treatment, he renewed his driver's license and had a new photo taken. I've seen that photo and other photos, pre- and post-treatment. He is a handsome man: rugged, nice eyes, a relaxed smile, friendly. But in the photo taken while he was undergoing chemo, his head is swollen to what looks to be 1.25 its normal size; his skin tone ranges from orange to red to white to bruised green; his eyes are nearly shut with the swelling. His face looks like the surface of Jupiter's moon Io, which used to be my favorite moon. Now Io looks to me like a nauseated chemotherapy patient. My friend's husband looks as if he is in a lot of pain in that picture. My friend tells me that her husband refuses to take a new post-chemo driver's license photo. Every now and then you read somewhere that some actor or some musician or some combination of the two is the essence of cool. You know what cool is? Using as photo evidence of your identity a picture of yourself taken in the middle of a round of brutal chemotherapy, surviving both cancer and chemotherapy, and recognizing that the photo is honestly you although it looks nothing like you now. That's cool.

In my experience with CLL/SLL so far, my only physical complaints have been persistent fatigue, a relatively mild discomfort that I'm sure I will look back on someday with fond memories, and some sort of strange acne. To have red bumps popping up in clusters all over my scalp, my face, and my neck at the age of fifty-nine makes me just want to whine, "For God's sake, I thought I was through with this at the end of puberty." I feel compelled to apologize for my unsightly scalp every time I get my hair cut. One product I've found over the counter does suppress the outbreaks as long as I have it on, always: benzoyl peroxide, which comes in a white paste. So to fight the strange acne I have chalky white splotches everywhere, including on my scalp, tangling up whatever hair I have left on top of my head.

I don't think either my oncologist or my dermatologist knows exactly what is responsible for the skin outbreaks. My guess is extra lymphatic fluid from my engorged lymph nodes, especially prominent in the neck and face, leaking to the surface and causing a histamine reaction. Those swollen lymph nodes are most obvious, when I am dressed, in my face and neck. I look like a chipmunk who somehow hasn't learned to store his food properly in his cheeks so that chunks keep slipping down his neck. Either that or a walking cubist-period Picasso portrait, all angles and protruding bits that don't fit, like an adult-skilled jigsaw puzzle mashed together by a frustrated child (or a happy child with no understanding of jigsaw puzzle rules).

I'm really too old to be vain about my appearance, and there was never much to be vain about even when I was young. Instead of those chili peppers that young attractive professors get on ratemyprofessors.com, I've been most recently compared by one clever student to a combination of Don Knotts and Forrest Gump. See, I hate to even mention this, because people who know me are now saying to themselves, "Oh, yeah, I see it. Yeah, that's right." And now they know that I check ratemyprof. When I was younger some people compared me to Christopher Walken (my face, not my voice, which is closer to that of Foghorn Leghorn), which shows you just how narrow the line is between the goofy grotesque and the scary grotesque.

Here's just how good I've got it right now. For the most part I have only annoying, embarrassing problems like acne and lots of time-consuming and body-invasive doctor appointments. I'll be seeing a dermatologist soon, who will no doubt take a magnifying glass to every square inch of my body, murmuring as she inspects my bumps and moles and various other imperfections. It's too late to get back in shape by lifting weights. I'm sure this will be a full-body manual scan. I'm too fatigued to lift weights, and even when I tried once recently, the lymph nodes in my armpits hurt and seemed to get in the way of free motion.

CLL/SLL puts one at a higher risk for many other cancers, so if a healthcare specialist can potentially find cancer, you pretty much need to hand your body over to that specialist for a really close look more frequently than most people are comfortable with. Among the extra physicians I have to allow to prod, probe, poke, examine, and look at me with alarming frequency are dermatologists, oncologists, pathologists, surgeons, general physicians, dentists (for oral cancer screenings), and gastroenterologists (who pretty much take the other end for examination in performing colonoscopies).

The only good thing about a colonoscopy, other than being cleared of colon cancer, which is not guaranteed, is Versed. If pre-operative fentanyl makes me an amateur comic, in my experience Versed makes me an amateur, if easily distracted and inept, Don Juan. I've had Versed only pre-colonoscopy, so it does present some complications in the wooing phase of my fleeting crushes on nurses. I've read that a recent developing trend in the colonoscopy world is to use propofol,[1] which may make procedures easier for gastroenterologists, but it would be difficult to woo my colonoscopy nurse when unconscious. I prefer Versed, because a colonoscopy is not really that painful anyway, except for the part where the gastroenterologist inflates my colon with CO_2 so he or she can have a good thorough look around a part of my body that really, I'd prefer to keep cloaked. Versed also makes me feel absolutely and endlessly in love with the world.

The last time I had a colonoscopy, the attending nurse held my left hand as she numbed the back of it for the insertion of the needle that would deliver the Versed. Once the Versed started flowing, and the gastroenterologist started his business, I instantly fell in love with my nurse. She talked to me to distract me from the pain, but it didn't matter what she said—I felt a surge of love for all living things as the Versed flowed through my bloodstream. At one point, I stroked her hand with my right hand as she held my left, mumbling, "You're so nice!" The gastroenterologist found one polyp, neatly clipped it off, and pronounced me pure as a December snowflake. The polyp was dutifully sent off to a pathologist for a closer look, but it was no surprise to anyone when the verdict of "benign" was returned a week later.

In recovery I somehow lost track of and interest in my colonoscopy nurse. I was still in love with life, though, and my attention shifted to two other nurses (one in training) who were to see me through recovery. I was feeling so good that really I saw nothing to recover from. My angels offered me some apple juice, which tasted like the finest mountain stream water flavored with apple concentrate. I drank two cartons quickly because I was so dehydrated that the skin on my arms looked like crunchy dried leaves ready to crumble if anyone bumped me too hard. By that time the nurses had allowed Heather to join me in recovery. They stood ready to hand me as many juice boxes as I wanted as Heather sat at the foot of the bed and said, "You look a little pale, but I guess that's normal." She comforted me by patting my foot, as I alternately stared at her face, thinking, "I love my wife; she's so nice!" and then stared at anything my out-of-focus eyeballs happened to stop on momentarily.

Looking at my leafy arms in wonder, I suddenly began to feel as if I were sinking through the bed, and then I slumped to my right side, lacking the energy even to keep my body upright. I slurred, "I don't feel very good at all," and both nurses and Heather, alarmed, called for help. A senior nurse walking by took one look at me and said, "He's vagaling down. He's got to fart." She shouted in a voice that was more an order than a warning, "Sir, you must fart! You are vagaling down." I knew about the vagus nerve, which extends to the abdomen, and that it is somehow involved in fainting, but I had no idea what the connection was to farting. I learned later that if there is too much CO_2 left in the colon, the colon can press against the vagus nerve and cause a drop in blood pressure and sudden loss of consciousness. At that moment, I felt ill, really ill, and was willing to try anything. But then I looked around: three nurses, my wife at the foot of the bed, and other patients in beds scattered around the room. I said, "I would, but . . ." and then gestured to everyone. The senior nurse barked, "Everybody out! Everybody out, now!" The two younger nurses and Heather left the area, and the senior nurse pulled the flimsy hospital bed curtain, which was so thin I could see though it, around my bed. I concentrated and then let loose the longest, loudest fart I've ever heard outside of a movie made for teenage boys. Then I perked right up and finished my third apple juice carton. I felt perfectly cloaked and in love with the world once again.

Heather Responds to
"Quit That Looking at Me"

I know all about fainting, although I'd never seen Don do it. I'm the fainter, as he has said. Years ago when we lived in Texas, we celebrated our anniversary by going out to one of those Texas steak houses where they just throw a big hunk of charcoaled meat at you along with a lot of other food like baked potatoes and beans, and even salad if you want it (but nobody ever wants it). We both stuffed ourselves and then went to see *Alien 3* because why not? I like scary movies and Sigourney Weaver's badass style.

About five minutes into the movie, there is a close-up of a giant hypodermic needle inching its way toward Sigourney's vein as they revive her from her crash landing. I turned to Don and said, "I don't think I can watch this. Tell me when the needle's gone." But the image is still in my head and I can't stop seeing it. I opened my eyes, saw dark spots, and I started feeling light-headed, a familiar sign that I'm about to faint. But I was also queasy. I told Don I didn't feel so good and was feeling faint. He said, "Do you want to leave? We can leave." I said I couldn't walk and that I was getting more nauseated by the minute. And then I found myself coming to.

Don said, "Heather, you just fainted. Your head fell on your chest. Do you want to leave? We need to get you out of here." It made me mad because I kept telling him I was going to faint and couldn't walk.

I fainted again, apparently, because he repeated pretty much what he had just said when I woke up the second time. This irritated me even more. I had never experienced this alternation between fainting and queasiness before and I remember wondering if I was having a stroke.

Days after the whole ordeal, Don told me that he hadn't known what to do so he just watched the movie with one eye and monitored my condition with the other. That sounded stupid to me at the time and still does. He was *watching the movie?* But, I suppose, what else was he going to do? Usually I come out of these fainting spells after one good loss of consciousness, and then everything is okay.

Well, the way he tells the story, it was lights out for me a third time. He's watching the movie, and this is the one in which the alien somehow gets itself inside a dog, and you know what's coming, and Don says that at the exact moment the dog explodes across the screen because the alien has burst out of it (as they are wont to do), I projectile-vomited (still unconscious) across three rows of seats in front of us. Apparently one of the frequent side effects of a vaso-vagal response is nausea. Until that day, this had never happened to me.

Luckily for me and everyone else, no one was sitting in those three rows in front of us.

Don said, "That's it. We're getting you out of here." And he pulled me up and helped me to the exit and to the car. We immediately rushed to an emergency room because I was sure I was having a stroke, and we spent three hours waiting for tests to be run and for an ER doctor to figure out what was going on.

His diagnosis: "You passed out due to a full stomach, bending over to keep from fainting, and then nausea occurred because the needle triggered a vagal vascular response." His suggestion: "Don't watch anymore bad movies." That made me laugh but kind of ticked me off too.

Yeah, so Don gets colonoscopy nurses who hang on his every fart, and I get an emergency room doctor who's a film critic.

Notes

1. Greenwald, "Sedation."

Where Did I Last See It?

September 13

HAVING CANCER MIGHT IMPROVE YOUR memory, if it's true what we hear about the exercise of memory functions increasing its capacity. These days I'm spending quite a bit of time trying to learn and remember what the dozens of available forms of chemotherapy are designed to do, what ZAP-70, 13q, and 17p deletions in the genetics of the white blood cell mean, portend, or prognose, and how different forms of chemotherapy interact with those genetics. I also have the mundane tasks of staying on top of the increase in WBC each month and, more important, how other cells are reacting to that crowding (counts of red blood cells and platelets, for example) from month to month. It's practically a part-time job just trying to make and keep all the appointments that are necessary: oncologist (once a month), dermatologist (every six months), family physician (every three months), surgeon (as needed), lab work (more times than I can count). I make notes before each appointment with Heather's help, to remind me of specific questions I have, mostly inspired by my reading. I'm hoping my various doctors see my questions arising from the proper level of paranoia. At my last oncologist visit, in August, I'd planned to ask him about ordering a PSA blood test, whether it was okay to try B12 for energy, and what he knew about ibrutinib trials.

The first thing they did at that visit was test the level of my WBC which, shockingly, turned out to be up 33 percent over the last month. Then followed palpation of lymph nodes (right axillary area larger), spleen, and liver, the latter two normal with no change in remaining lymph node areas visible beneath the skin. The rise in WBC level confirmed for my oncologist that he wanted to continue to monitor me closely by seeing me each month. In July the rise had been only 7 percent. Learning the news of a 33 percent rise in August (I had been hoping for at least a leveling of WBC), quite honestly I panicked, closing my eyes and disappearing into my mind to calculate the alarming compound interest over a period of perhaps just three more months. When I emerged and opened my eyes again, I had to look at my notes to remember my questions about PSA, B12, and ibrutinib, realizing now that maybe I wasn't being paranoid enough.

I'm lucky but not surprised that Heather wants me to live as long as I can. She's so worried that she takes off work to go with me to oncology appointments now, not just to hold my hand (although I have to admit she does) but mainly to serve as my backup memory. There is so much to remember under pressure, especially when something like an unexpected 33 percent increase in WBC in one month takes your breath away. Her interpretation usually puts a more positive spin on what the oncologist says than mine, but not always. Just yesterday she told me that the oncologist has been subtly suggesting for two appointments now that I shouldn't hope for ibrutinib (a relatively nontoxic treatment) as a first treatment because the trials for ibrutinib as a first response are only a couple of years under way and won't conclude for several more years. Me, I was convinced that my oncologist had told us that approval was perhaps as little as two years out. Subsequent Internet reading on current trials supports the interpretation of closer to ten years for potential approval (see "Afterward" for news on this that I don't think any of us expected: Heather, me, or my oncologist). I've read in more than one place that if you have a serious illness, it is wise to take a friend or family member with you to appointments, especially if you are occasionally a bit absentminded like me.

Not that I am an absentminded professor. That stereotype elicits images of some goof who might forget to wear pants on any given day, although I did once witness a professor lecture for seventy-five minutes with her sweater turned inside out. My absentmindedness is endemic not to my job but at all levels of my life.

I was an absentminded child. In elementary school I would regularly walk into the wrong classes at the wrong time of day. "Lost again, Donny?" the teacher would ask. Some children laughed. Most looked at me as if I were crazy. No one just walks into the wrong class. At a university where I used to work, when I lived close enough that I sometimes walked to my office, twice I had to walk home just because I could not find my car in the parking lot. I simply forgot where I parked. At 7:00 a.m. the following morning my car stood out like a sign reading, "Here's your car, dummy!"

And it does no good to ask me where I last saw my keys or my wallet or my car, even though Heather always does ask. If I *knew* where I last saw them, they wouldn't be lost. Furthermore, I don't trust my keys or wallet or anything else (well, except maybe my car) to stay in the same place I left them. I have cats who like nothing better than to swat objects like pens, pencils, keys, and glasses under sofas and chairs. I wish I could blame them for losing track of my car too.

Back when I had panic/anxiety disorder for a couple of years, I was a compulsive checker. You know: fires out, door locked, cats inside (although they never go out), lights off. My psychologist at the time told me I needed to be more mindful. That is, I needed to be consciously present when I locked the door. I believed him then; I don't now. If I wanted to be consciously present for every damned thing I do all day long, I'd have to be stoned on some pretty good weed—all day long, as in "Yeah, that door is locked. Yep, locked. I just saw myself do it. Yep, I just thought about just seeing myself do it. Okay, where's my car?" I don't know about other people, but I stopped being a compulsive checker when I stopped being compulsive, not when I became more mindful. Now I lock the door and just don't think about it again. If there were a sign halfway between my house and my office that asked, "Did you lock your house door when you left?" I would probably turn right back around and check.

Heather Responds to "Where Did I Last See It?"

It is true that with the cancer diagnosis, we find it hard to keep up with the flood of incoming information. We absorb it, but it sometimes takes time for one or both of us to process the information, and then there are always the disagreements about what some particular doctor said, in spite of notes that we both take. I'm usually better at taking notes, probably for two reasons: (1) I'm not the one who has the cancer, and (2) I'm a compulsive note taker, which helps in my job as a university administrator. A rare counterexample: Don has been forbidden by his oncologist to eat salad at restaurants or sushi anywhere. There's too much threat of nasty microorganisms taking advantage of his impaired immune system. Don insists that the oncologist said no salad at restaurants or sushi "until you are through chemotherapy and recovery." I insist that he said, "Never, ever, from this point forward." Given all the other information that we are attempting to process, the question of salad and sushi seems low priority, and it is. In spite of several opportunities, we have yet to remember to ask Don's oncologist to settle the disagreement. Much later it turned out that Don was right on this one.

The Evanescence
of the Epidermis

September 16

H EATHER CAME WITH ME to my most recent dermatology
appointment because (1) the dermatologist wanted to rule
out any melanomas as melanoma is a bad cancer to have in itself,
but in conjunction with leukemia it sounds horrifying; (2) as usual
there were lots of questions to ask and answers to keep track of
because the most annoying side effect I have now, beside the
fatigue, is adult acne and rashes; and (3) Heather and my dermatologist are friends, or let's say, they know one another so well that
they are on a first-name basis.

The assistant to the dermatologist takes blood pressure,
oxygen levels, pulse—for what reason I don't know. Then she
orders me to disrobe to my underwear, no socks. I expected this,
but I also expected a paper gown. When I ask for one, she tells
me, "Most men prefer to just sit in their underwear. But if you
want one . . ." And she opens a cabinet and points to stacks of
gowns. I say, "No, if I get cold, I know where they are." It's hot in
the room anyway. I'm already sweating through my plaid boxers
and through the white paper that looks like butcher paper and am
sticking to the Naugahyde of the examination chair like a baby
with a damp butt and moles.

Doctor comes in, hail-fellow-well-met greets Heather, looks
me in the eye, and says, "Hey, stranger. Haven't seen you in a

while." Last time I saw her she shaved a mole (non-cancerous) frozen with nitrogen off my stomach. I had forgotten how attractive this doctor is. I tell the attractive doctor the full story of the CLL/SLL battle and say I want a thorough checkup and would really appreciate something to take care of the acne and the rashes. She starts peering through what looks like a lighted jeweler's loupe at the top of my scalp, examining everything, every mole, every imperfection, with what appears to be 20x magnification. She checks behind my ears, in my ears, under my arms ("nice scars"), chest, abdomen, back, legs, bottom of feet, between toes. There's only one thing she's worried about, a two-toned mole on the back of my left leg, which she says we ought to biopsy. Heather has been jotting notes about two-toned moles and biopsies and length of time for results of biopsy and so on when the doctor turns to her and asks, "Any moles or other marks in the penis or scrotal area?"

For some reason it doesn't immediately occur to me that it's somewhat strange that the attractive doctor has been talking to me exclusively during the lengthy full-body search but then turns to Heather for information about my penis and scrotal area. Before the thought has time to cross my mind that hey, I know my penis and scrotal area at least as well as Heather, maybe better, my wife answers, "Yes. He has a mole." I start pulling my underwear down just far enough, but no farther, for the doctor to see the mole. But I can't find the mole, although I thought I knew exactly where it was. The doctor asks me to pull down my underwear all the way, so I comply and then start assiduously trying to remember everything I know about baseball. Heather gets up, comes around me from behind, and with her index finger jabs exactly where I thought the mole was. She says, "It's right there!" Jab. The doctor takes her 20x lighted magnification loupe and asks, "Where?" At this point I'm bent over with my head upside down, all three of us staring directly at my penis area, searching desperately for a mole that is supposed to be there but isn't. And then I remember that I had that mole removed four years ago by a dermatologist in another state. I mumble something like, "Maybe that's one my last dermatologist removed."

Obviously I'm not to be trusted anymore, so the doctor performs a thorough examination of my penis and scrotal area without my direction. She finds nothing of interest.

The doctor's assistant numbs the area on my leg with the two-toned mole, and the doctor neatly excises it with a curved razor blade, cauterizes the wound, and bandages it. I make another appointment six months out because melanomas can pretty much pop up almost overnight. Leaving, I turn to the doctor and thank her, using her professional title—"Doctor." She says, "Please call me ——," her first name. Given how well she now knows every inch of my body, I think, paradoxically, that I might rather stick to "Doctor." I don't know. Everything's so complicated.

**Heather Responds to
"The Evanescence of the Epidermis"**

Honestly, I was as startled as Don when the dermatologist asked me if there were any moles in the penis or scrotal area. I thought fleetingly and flippantly, "How the hell should I know?" But I couldn't say that to a physician. You could say that maybe about, oh, the bottom of the feet or the areas between the toes or even the area behind the ears. Who looks at the bottom of anyone's feet or between their toes or behind their ears? I'm not sure I'd recognize a significant change in the bottom of my own feet for weeks. But you don't ask, "How should I know?" about your husband's penile and scrotal areas. That might imply something. The implications are wide open to too many different, perhaps even conflicting, interpretations. Was I supposed to say: "How the hell would I know? I haven't looked at his dick in months!" Or: "How the hell would I know? I see it every day, but I don't *examine* it." And why ask me anyway? Even if I had observed a change that Don hadn't noticed for some reason, like perhaps because he sometimes doesn't notice even the most obvious things, such as whether we are running low on toilet paper or paper towels or coffee or if the house is on fire, wouldn't I have told Don: "Hey, dude, your dick has a mole in the exact shape of Texas on it. Did you know that?" That would be hard to ignore, even for Don. So if there had been a change, I would have mentioned it to Don, and he would have known.

The information overload and attendant stress explain why neither of us remarked on the strange interaction in the dermatologist's examining room for at least two weeks. We were in fact in the waiting area for an oncology appointment when Don asked, "Wasn't that strange when the dermatologist asked you whether there were any changes to my quote penile or scrotal areas end quote?" Then I thought about it and laughed until tears ran down my face as I remembered all the things that had run through my mind at the time. We both laughed and repeated the conversation two or three times, like a joke that never gets old, ever.

Make a Wish

I'M NOT YET AT THE STAGE where (if I were nine) people would be offering to take me to Disneyland. Fulfilling a dying child's wish to meet a famous pop star, famous athlete, or even a famous mouse seems unquestionably to be a kind thing to do. It has been so long since I was a kid I have no conception of what impending death might mean to someone who has barely begun to live. When I was a kid I thought that a year stretched beyond our sight line of imagination. I was eight when Kennedy was assassinated in Dallas, maybe about 50 miles from where I was sleepwalking through the third grade. When my teacher announced that the president had been shot, I thought to myself, "Big deal! I get shots every year." Nobody in my young baby boomer life ever really got "*shot* shot." My grandfather was the first to die in my family, of a heart attack. I was seven. I cried at the funeral because I thought I was supposed to.

I have absolutely no idea when I developed a sense of personal mortality, but it must have occurred sometime between ages ten and twenty-five. My only memorable mortality anxiety developed in my late twenties, when I began to fly airlines fairly regularly. During that time Heather lived and taught in Denton, Texas, while I was in Houston in graduate school. I'd fly up every two weeks to spend the weekend, and each flight was torture, from takeoff to landing—sweaty palms, rapid pulse, muscle-cramping grip on both armrests. The flight was mercifully short, about forty minutes, but during those years I had recurrent nightmares in which planes I was on crashed or nearly crashed or flew too low or had to use freeways as emergency landing runways.

The fear became so intense that I took the bus from Houston to Dallas—once. I bought a one-way airline ticket to return. That bus ride, lasting approximately fourteen hours, cured me of ever taking a bus between Houston and Dallas, primarily through its numbing boredom, relieved only by stopping to pick up approximately twenty newly released convicts from the state penitentiary at Huntsville. Although they were all well behaved (a virtue probably beaten into them in prison), they all sounded intentionally or even ironically overly polite, talking among themselves or to other passengers or to the bus driver, who would unpredictably occasionally snap at them as if they were still prisoners. The only one I met who would say anything to my twenty-something self other than "Yes, sir" and "No, sir" complained that he was supposed to check in with his parole officer in Fort Worth in the morning and stay with his mother that night, "but fuck that shit 'cause I'm going to get me a woman and some liquor." Most of the others probably had plans just as interesting, but they weren't going to share them with a civilian.

To survive cancer you're supposed to have goals. You're supposed to have something to live for. One way to do that at my age might be to make a bucket list of things I haven't done: (1) move to Mexico, (2) rob a bank, (3) get hooked on heroin, (4) kill a bad guy while saving a friend in a drug deal gone bad. No doubt this narrative would give me a reason to live and certainly take my mind off the disease. But none of these things is likely to happen because I don't want them to happen and because I'd have to give up the extraordinarily lucky life that I live now.

I have a life that fits me remarkably well. It's quiet, with two cats, a dog, a wife whom I love, a few friends whom I love. I like most aspects of my job, especially teaching and writing, in that order. I'm lucky. If someone asked me to make a wish, I honestly don't know what it would be beyond, obviously, taking away the unwelcome guest in my life, which is literally impossible, given current treatment options. I'm old enough not to wish for the impossible.

When I was in therapy for panic disorder for a couple of years, the psychologist I went to was a brilliant communicator. I know this because usually I don't listen to anyone at any time about anything, but he eventually got through to me. The misery of panic disorder also probably motivated me to listen more closely than I normally do.

My thoughts all day, every day, for two years were dominated by hypothetical scenarios such as, "Maybe I hit somebody on a bicycle with my truck on my way to the appointment today. I went around the block twice, but I didn't see anyone injured. But I came way too close to that guy on the bicycle. Maybe I hit him." Or, "What if I plagiarized someone else whose work I read in doing research for my manuscript and just forgot that I read that person?" This latter fear ate up hours and hours and days and days of my time: I went to the library to track down books and articles, sometimes through interlibrary loan, that sometimes I had actually read but sometimes hadn't even seen before but imagined that I had read. Or, "What if I somehow unintentionally plagiarized myself?" leading me to the worst punishment, rereading everything I had ever published, comparing each document line by line with my new manuscript. Or, "What if in cleaning out files, I threw out for recycling Heather's invaluable research notes from years before on the American Indian language that she studied?" This last obsession entailed opening box after box of research notes that Heather had packed away and checking with her to make absolutely sure that all of her notes were indeed still where she had stored them. People who live with victims of panic disorder suffer as well.

My psychologist explained over and over that for some combination of reasons, mainly due to faulty brain circuitry, exacerbated by two job moves to two new universities in less than three years, and partially due to my father's own battle with cancer, which included periodic stays in hospice care, I was under more stress than I was used to coping with and my stress reactor was over-reacting, inventing imaginary problems to solve. He explained, perhaps ten times, "Think of it as a bucket of stress. It's full. You cannot allow yourself to put anything more in, at least until you take something else out. You are obsessing on stressful imaginary scenarios as if in imagining them you can control them." Once he even drew a diagram to illustrate his point. It stayed on his white-board for weeks. I heard the words, and I remembered them some-times, and some of those times those words helped calm me down and stopped me from continuing on with some new fantasy, such as that I had perhaps caused the cardiomyopathy that killed one of my dogs years ago.

My psychologist was, for good reason, not above losing patience with me occasionally when the bucket metaphor didn't seem to be getting through. One day, he said, "Okay, I'll use lan-guage you can understand. You're a linguist, right?"

"Right."

"You study language. How it's constructed? How it works?"

"Right."

"This 'What if?' that you get caught up in... that's bad for you. Don't conjugate that verb."

"Excuse me?"

"Whenever you start thinking, 'What if this?' or 'What if that?' or 'What if the next thing?' don't... conjugate... that... verb! Can you remember that?"

"Yeah, I can remember that."

I use that command to this day to stop my sometimes mildly obsessional thoughts: "Don't conjugate that verb!" stops me in my obsessive linguistic tracks. Words to live by.

I understand the bucket metaphor as well, now that I'm calm enough to think about it. It is actually the most useful metaphor my psychologist has ever given me as a tool. Everyone experiences stress; stress is not even necessarily a bad thing. But having too many things in your stress bucket is bad and counterproductive. Manage your stress bucket. Do not overfill it.

As for that other bucket metaphor, a bucket list, my goal is not to have one. A bucket list is about the future. Whenever I think about a bucket list, it's just one more obsessive thought to add to my stress bucket. Who needs a bucket of buckets? There will never be enough time to do everything in life that I would want to do, even given almost unlimited time. Thus, the only time that is satisfyingly real and satisfyingly achievable is now. I think of real, achievable time as that time that can be paid attention to and enjoyed rather than worried over—that it will come too fast and pass even more rapidly.

All the doctors—family physician, surgeon, oncologist—who either initially diagnosed or confirmed CLL/SLL said exactly the same thing, as if a cancer diagnosis came with numbered instructions on what to say to the patient: "Go home and live your life normally," which is some of the most paradoxical advice I've ever received. It's like "Don't conjugate the 'verb' 'What if?'" You couldn't even if you wanted to. But if you try, and you should, you'll realize that there can be a peace and even euphoria in owning an empty bucket.

Heather Responds to
"Make a Wish"

I don't know how Don would make a bucket list even if he wanted to. To have a bucket list, you pretty much have to have a set of consistent goals. And Don is the most changeable person I've ever known, from what he eats to what he reads to what he watches on TV. I refer to what Don is currently eating as what he is "on," as in "Are you still on salads?" or "Are you still on grilled cheese sandwiches?" because he will eat the same thing day after day for months at a time until he's suddenly off ravioli or off nuts or whatever it is, with no explanation at all. I'll just discover six unopened cans of nuts gathering dust in the pantry and have to ask, "Are you off nuts now?" as if he's just kicked a crack addiction. So if skydiving were on his bucket list, were he to make one and be able to find it, it would end up that he's just jumped out of the airplane for the umpteenth time and decided halfway down he doesn't want to do that anymore.

The two years that he was suffering from anxiety disorder were the worst. They were worse than the couple of months that we've been dealing with his cancer diagnosis, and worse even than his bouts with depression. I think he agrees. That may sound odd. But to put anxiety disorder in context, in the middle of the two years of his severe anxiety, we tried to get extra life insurance for Don, but he was turned down by the insurance company because anxiety disorder is associated with an increased risk for suicide. So it's not as if cancer is necessarily worse because it carries a higher likelihood for death. And the symptoms of the anxiety attacks are nearly as disabling as the promised side effects of the chemotherapy that he is yet to be treated with.

And I think I did say that Don rides motorcycles. When he picked up that hobby again, against my wishes, I insisted that we get extra life insurance for him. This was long before the anxiety attacks. Motorcycling is one of the few hobbies besides fishing that he's stuck with over the years. He rides his motorcycle to go fishing, thus insisting on making fishing dangerous too. And he carries a gun. I'm surprised that he doesn't have a bucket list that includes snake handling, base jumping, or anything else that carries an increased risk of mortality. So, yeah, he's all Zen about not having a bucket list because basically if he had a bucket list he'd have to commit himself to it, no matter what goofy thing was on the list. And there's always some new goofy thing that is more attractive than yesterday's enthusiasm.

You're the Expert:
So Listen to Me Carefully

October 11

M Y PRIMARY TEST for whether a person is an asshat or a decent human being is whether that person listens as well as speaks. Some people do nothing but speak—these are the asshats. Some both listen and speak. Few simply listen. The thoughts coming from inside our heads are constantly banging against the walls of our skulls and demanding exit. I almost certainly talk too much in the presence of students in my job. Part of this disorder comes with the job. A professor, contrary to a lot of current educational faddishness, is paid to communicate knowledge and passion for that knowledge. It's very difficult to do that if all you do is listen. But if you don't listen, you'll have absolutely no idea whether your students understand a topic, what excites them or painfully bores them, or what they imagine a certain career to be like. That would make you, or me, an asshat professor. On the website ratemyprofessors.com, in addition to the chili peppers for the hot young assistant professors and admittedly some of the still-smoking-hot associate and full professors (there are such blessed creatures), I think there should be an asshat GIF image. Why not?

I've had periodic reservations about the judgment of some of my physicians, mainly because I sometimes get the feeling from them that they are not listening to me. Some of them talk but don't listen. Some of them answer questions but only the questions that they want you to have asked. My six-foot-plus surgeon lost his six-foot-plus temper with me once before my first shoulder surgery when I questioned him about when I could get back to skiing and bicycling; it was the third time I'd asked because he seemed not to hear the question the first two times. He said, "I'm the surgeon, and you have to trust me, and you have to make getting well your first priority by physical therapy." I looked at his attending nurse with an expression on my face that said, "Who is this asshat?" Her expression answered, "This is your hand in this card game. Either play it or walk away from the table." In this case I just ended up doing what I felt like when I felt up to it (clearing it first with my physical therapists) and didn't bother my surgeon with questions like that anymore. Just like when I was a kid, I knew better than to ask my parents whether I could smoke or play with matches. I just did it. My surgeon and I got on famously once I stopped asking for his permission to do anything. I'd recommend him to anyone. The difference between my surgeon and my oncologist is that my surgeon wasn't trying to save my life. He merely made it worth living by removing an enormous burden of pain using his expertise in drilling, scraping, and cutting. I love the guy. No, really, I do. He's handsome, tall, super smart, very funny, and kind to boot. Just don't ask him a question that really means something like, "When is all this annoying surgery and recovery business going to be over so that I can get back to my life?"

Psychiatrists, unlike some surgeons, really need to be skilled listeners. I've fired more than one psychiatrist for being a horrible listener. One was obsessively convinced that I was bipolar. Every two weeks he would begin our session with the standard questions for bipolar diagnosis.

"Do you sometimes talk too much or too fast or too loud?"

"No."

"You've said that you have depression and anxiety, but do you sometimes feel or act manic?"

"No."

"Have you made any irrational large purchases recently?"

I hesitated on this one because I wondered whether paying for psychiatry—not cheap—was irrational, especially with this guy. "No, I don't think so."

"Do you laugh at inappropriate moments?"

"No."

I asked Heather to observe one session. She noted that the psychiatrist changed his instructions to me approximately every five minutes on medication recommendation and dosage as well as on frequency of treatment. She was unable to take coherent notes because he changed his mind on practically everything at least once. She noticed that he answered his cell phone twice during our session, which I had missed. Her conclusion afterward: "Your psychiatrist is bipolar." I asked around town, and it turned out this psychiatrist was known for pushing bipolar diagnoses and inappropriate medication on his patients.

There is, so far as I can tell, no clinically tested cure for CLL/SLL. Once you get the disease, you eventually die from it or with it. Of more concern to me now is that I'm beginning to suspect that my oncologist and I are having communication problems, and that bothers me—a lot—because I think it's my fault.

He palpates my nodes and asks about night sweats and the other symptoms of advanced-stage leukemia, but he steadfastly refuses to prognose either my survival time or even when I am likely to enter chemotherapy (because he has "been wrong on both sides of the estimates too many times"). I fully realize the nature of statistical likelihood. It doesn't bother me that he doesn't want to prognose. Apparently I'm going to have to be more direct about what I'm really concerned about. I've been indirect thus far, I suppose, because I don't want to appear scared. It's a kind of pride that has kept me from saying straight out what I mean. I want to be the kind of person who appears to be fearless in the presence of both cancer and its treatment.

What I really want to know is whether he realizes that the

prospect of chemotherapy is about the most frightening thing I can think of now. I like being alive. I don't want to die. But I don't fear death, or at least I don't think I do. I want to put chemotherapy off for as long as it is safe to do so, even if that involves walking around with a pustular head and face and lymph nodes that look like I've been eating rocks and have several of them caught in my pharynx. Chemotherapy itself can cause cancer—not in all cases but in enough to frighten the average patient. Chemo can make you throw up, ruin your appetite, cause your hair to fall out, and create painful mouth sores. And yes, I also realize that these side effects of treatment are mere statistical likelihoods, but they scare me witless. When I told my dental hygienist that I had CLL/SLL but wasn't expecting to enter chemotherapy anytime soon, she told me to buy a special mouthwash that has no alcohol in it, the reason being that chemotherapy attacks cells that reproduce rapidly, not just cancer cells but cells like those that line the inside of our mouths. And alcohol in mouthwash exacerbates that problem. I was shocked and dismayed that she simply assumed that I would be entering chemotherapy soon enough for it to be prudent to order the special mouthwash right away.

I'm going to have to beat down my pride at my next appointment with my oncologist and be honest about what I want to know. I haven't been honest, I think, because I haven't been listening to myself, haven't been listening to my real fears at this point in the progression of my cancer.

In my academic field of linguistics, opinions from speakers of a language about their language are nearly always revealing of something interesting about the structure or social function of language. Therefore, linguists are trained above all to listen, because in listening one learns not only the structure of the language but also the social attitudes that surround it.

I once took a motorcycle trip from Illinois to Texas. It was a great trip, one that I would happily repeat. I took mostly county roads. I wasn't in a hurry. I stopped to eat at filling stations/diners that made fresh ham sandwiches like I remember from the local grocery store when I was a kid. Once I got near Texas, beat up by the rain and the bugs and the dirt, I chose to explore an area I'd never been to, the extreme northeastern piney woods corner of Texas, right below Arkansas. I stopped in a town named DeKalb, Texas, because I was living then in DeKalb, Illinois. At a gas station I struck up a conversation with the woman running the cash register.

"You know, I'm from a town in Illinois with the exact same name as this one here where we are."

"Oh, yeah, I know about that town. That's where you all got all that corn."

"Yep. Lots of corn. How do you pronounce the name of this town here, because I think they might pronounce it different up in Illinois?"

"Oh, yeah, up there, they say 'DEEkahb,' like the corn."

"Yep, that's how they do it."

"Here, we say 'DEEkab.'"

"DEEkab?"

"Yep, the *k* is silent. If you don't say it right, the schoolteachers will correct you."

If you're a linguist or familiar with a north Texas accent, you can probably decode the rough spelling pronunciation that I've given the woman's attempts to represent an Illinois accent and then the right accent in her part of Texas (including the interesting vowel differences in the second syllable). This conversation richly illustrates not only linguistic behavior but attitude. Everybody who speaks a language is a natural-born linguist. And if we don't know a rule, we'll make it up, like the silent *k*, which is of course not silent at all. It's the *l* that disappears in the woman's attempts at both an Illinois pronunciation and a Texas pronunciation. She's wrong about the Illinois pronunciation, but *wrong* is not the right word. She is, above all, interesting as a human speaker of a language, with strong attitudes about what is right and what is wrong. I wouldn't dream of correcting her. And I wouldn't dream of not listening.

I'm sure some physicians tire of amateurs walking in with their self-diagnoses and self-prognoses freshly half-baked from the Internet. And I'm sure that patients lie quite a bit, even disguising their greatest fears. But if physicians and patients don't listen both to each other and to themselves, they'll miss the best parts of their relationship, chances to attend to the ephemeral consciousness that rises on the wisp of biochemical reactions, a connection that no one, and I mean no one, yet understands.[1] There is even the possibility that we will never be able to understand it, because how can a biochemical brain understand an emergent experience that has produced precious few words to describe itself? It is as hard to describe what it feels like to be alive—even using the word *alive*—as it is to describe what chocolate smells like, even using the word *chocolate*. And how interesting is that?

Heather Responds to
"You're the Expert: So Listen to Me Carefully"

Well, I don't want to pretend to be the expert here, but I'm not so sure that Don's biggest fear is the chemotherapy. Note that Don ends this entry with a meditation on how elusive the words used to describe *life* are and how elusive life itself is. One of Don's and my favorite books many, many years ago was Ernest Becker's *Denial of Death*.[2] We both read it several times and talked about it together and with a fellow academic and friend who found it especially interesting. Becker's thesis is that an enormous amount of human culture and human effort is directed at combating our fear of death—or, more specifically, the fear of a meaningless life. When fear is understood that way, it is hard to imagine anyone not being afraid of death unless that fearless person believes deeply in a religious orthodoxy that provides a predetermined overall goal and purpose for life and the afterlife.

Take your pick of dogmas. There are plenty. I think Don has

flirted with Jesus, especially since he's spent a good portion of his academic writing career trying to figure out the narrative tricks of that quirkiest of Catholic and southern writers, Flannery O'Connor. Don has never wanted to admit it, but I think you have to have some of the Jesus fever in you to appreciate O'Connor's fiction.

He's said that he's "done with O'Connor," although he's got one more paper in him, apparently, on the influence of somebody or other on her writing.

He also says he's turning his attention toward less literary subjects, but what is he doing? Writing a book (not this one, another one) on the self. *Self*, as he has told me himself, is nothing other than a secular code word for *soul*. Every time he turns around, he's looking for meaning in life. So do I believe him when he says that he's not afraid of death? Absolutely not. At least in the Ernest Becker sense of fear of a meaningless life.

A person who spends as much time as Don does writing and reading and torturing himself with self-doubt and anxiety has to be afraid of a meaningless life. And what would bring on such fear more strongly than this brush with mortality at a relatively young age? He has had friends die already, it's true, but none of those deaths has hit him hard because they were friends from twenty and thirty years ago. His father lived to be ninety; his mother is in her eighties. I think Don thought he had plenty of time to create a meaningful life. I think his problem is that he already has a meaningful life. He just hasn't read it carefully enough yet.

Notes

1. Harris, *Waking Up.*
2. Becker, *The Denial of Death.*

I'm Listening—for Now

October 22

MY LYMPH NODES have entered an overly enthusiastic growth spurt just in the last two and a half weeks, starting about ten days before my most recent appointment with my oncologist. I estimate that the visible ones doubled in size during that ten days. I was thinking seriously of buying a turtleneck sweater to hide the ones in my neck and under my chin, but then I thought it would be too much like a comb-over—too obvious, certainly to me and to people who knew that I had cancer. Most people overtly avoid noticing the swelling, which I appreciate, all except Heather, who is alarmed by the swelling and said so, which I also appreciate. The swelling, which has also increased in my groin nodes, helps explain some mysterious aches and pains I've been having. I'd noticed that my gait had slowed for no discernible reason other than what I thought to be pure fatigue. It turns out that the larger the nodes in the groin became, the more obvious was the pain at the extreme of my stride. I have been unconsciously slowing my gait to avoid the pain.

I suspected that my oncologist would be making the decision to put me in chemotherapy soon. He had said in an earlier appointment that I would have a month or two lead time from any decision that it was time to start chemotherapy to the actual beginning.

The first thing that always happens when I am seated in an examining room at my oncologist's office is that a nurse takes a blood sample to run through the blood panel analyzer. The procedure is remarkably easy: the nurse uses a clicking blade that cuts the skin on a finger just enough to draw blood, which the nurse then sucks into what looks like tiny eye droplet dispensers. The first few times a nurse drew blood I didn't even notice the almost imperceptible pain, but the combination of the audible click and the nick has me flinching every time now.

This time when my oncologist walked in with the blood results, he had a big smile on his face and said that my white blood cell count had dropped by 15,000, a good sign that perhaps the leukemia was going to hover for a while in a semi-stable state. But when I pulled my shirt aside and he got a look at my toadlike face and neck, he said, "Oh," and his face fell. After palpating the nodes, all of which had swollen, my oncologist said, "We are going to have to start chemotherapy soon." He excused himself and left the room for what I imagined at the time was a quick consult with his colleagues but later realized might just as easily have been a quick consult with the scheduler for chemotherapy.

That schedule is remarkably complex because you can have only so many people in the infusion room at a time. There are only so many seats for patients, and on any given day there are only so many nurses available to tend to patients. And those patients are by the nature of their treatment demanding of time.

It turns out that my oncologist had left the room also to schedule the surgery for a second biopsy and the installation of a subdermal chemotherapy port. My first day of treatment would involve changing the infusion bags that feed the port in my chest eight times.

Allow me to back up a minute and say, because I just remembered it, that after my oncologist said, "We are going to have to start chemotherapy soon," I starting crying, trying to suck air as I felt it being pulled from my chest by the panic. This was the real thing. I said, "Sorry, Doctor, it's just that it's a relief. I've been afraid of this so long, and now we're going to start doing something about the cancer. It's a good thing. I'm sorry." He patted me on the knee and gave me a reassuring squeeze as he left to call the surgeon and talk to the chemotherapy scheduler. I apologized for weeping, but I now think he probably sees this reaction a lot.

While he was gone I had more trouble catching my breath than stopping crying. I couldn't keep the air in my chest. It felt as if the air I was sucking in wasn't feeding my body, so my body rejected it quickly and just as quickly tried to suck in another chestful. Panic, I think, is what most people call this reaction.

The doctor came back into the room, sat down, and said, "So yes, we will begin chemotherapy as soon as possible."

"How soon?" I asked.

"Monday the 27th."

"Of this month?"

"Yes, of this month. The enlargement of your lymph nodes to this degree is a sign that we should have you enter treatment as soon as possible. The variation in the white blood cell count is normal. But I can't explain the sudden enlargement of your lymph nodes. That is odd for CLL/SLL. So we're going to have to do another biopsy to see whether the lymphoma has mutated."

Among the possible mutations is what is called Richter's transformation, which results in a rapid increase in the size of the lymph nodes and which is also very resistant to treatment of any kind. Median survival after diagnosis of Richter's transformation is eight to twelve months. Two facts argue against a diagnosis of the dreaded Richter's transformation or even the almost as dreaded 17p deletion at this point: usually in Richter's the lymph nodes increase in size in one area, and transformations normally do not occur this rapidly, just four months after diagnosis of CLL/SLL.[1] If anything, in my case, the lymph node swelling is spreading. The upper halves of both of my pectoral muscles actually protrude now because of increased swelling of the lymph nodes that lie directly under them on top of the rib cage.

I've been declaring for months that the scariest thing about having CLL/SLL is the chemotherapy. It was the worst thing in my imagination and now—hey presto—I no longer fear it. Until the ballooning of the nodes, I was spending a fair amount of time trying to work up the courage to tell my oncologist how frightened I was of chemotherapy, hoping that he would reassure me about the side effects and dangers. Now I'm more scared of these out-of-control lymph nodes, which if left untreated can swell large enough to cause strokes or heart failure by pressing on veins, arteries, or nerves leading to or away from the heart or brain. I've never gone to war, never been in battle, but I think that there is perhaps one way the metaphor of battling cancer might be appropriate. You might think you couldn't possibly be more afraid than you are of the machine guns strafing your entrenched position— until the enemy starts lobbing exploding shells toward you as well. War is hell, and so is cancer. In both cases the enemy is trying to kill you in more than one way, and in both cases only one side can win. Meaning one side dies.

If I have any consistency, it is inconsistency. Heather tells me that my ever-changing opinions on questions as basic as my favorite food or whether there is an afterlife of any significance make me one of the most interesting people she knows. The general cultural expectation of consistency is reflected even in what is fashionably called "learning modes," an educational fad that has now made its way into routine questions asked on intake to hospitals. When I went in for the second biopsy and the installation of a chemotherapy port in my chest, my intake nurse actually asked me how I learn best: by reading, listening, or doing. I briefly considered the appeal of learning how to install my own chemotherapy port by doing. Honestly, I didn't know how to answer the question, which I think the nurse was a bit embarrassed to have to ask in the first place, because I don't know how I learn best, or at least I don't think the choices of reading, listening, or doing adequately express my learning style. I thought for a minute and said, "I learn best by making mistakes, by being wrong," although in a more guarded moment I might have confidently declared that I learn best by listening.

The nurse didn't blink, but she also didn't check any of the available boxes on her intake sheet. She scribbled something in the margin, probably something along the lines of "smartass." Or maybe "asshat."

I don't mind making mistakes, and I'm not terribly ashamed of making them either. Arguing for my sometimes oddball positions frequently strengthens my resolve. The closer I get to sixty, the less disturbing it seems to be to have strong opinions on, say, what is to be done with my body once I'm dead, whether that death comes soon or many years from now. Right now I'm pretty convinced that if I get the chance shortly before I die, I want to get my first and last tattoo on my chest over my heart, one that says simply, "Have some damned respect, people!" Heather insists on considering this request rationally and points out with characteristically annoying logic that with my current compromised immune system, I am unlikely to be able to get any tattoo at all. I figure if my dog and two cats can be snuck in for final hugs and good-byes—and that's non-negotiable—I can get a tattoo artist smuggled in. I want this tattoo, a temporary henna tattoo if necessary, because I want to leave my body for some medical student or group of students to learn anatomy by systematically taking it apart. I'm guessing my tattoo will make the rumored disrespect among the very young for the dead either much better or much worse, perhaps the latter when the students reinstall my dissected brain stem directly to my lower colon, a crude metaphor but also an undeniably strong statement about the rights of the living over the dead.

After the local medical school students are done with me, I want to be cremated and my cremains scattered around the backyard of the house where Heather, my dog Lyle, my two cats Lamar and Lyndon, and I now live. I've told Heather that I want my ashes mixed with those of Bowie and Travis, two of our animals who have passed on now, and that eventually I'd like Lyle's ashes scattered there too and that I'd like her to get another dog after Lyle dies. Heather is currently treating this as yet another oddball opinion that I will change again at some point, probably sooner rather than later. I've listened to her (for me, irrelevant) arguments, for example, (1) that I won't know the new dog, and (2) that in any case being scattered in the backyard guarantees that my remains will be shat and pissed on by first Lyle and second Heather's next dog if she follows my wishes. What she doesn't understand is that I've already thought of these objections but to my mind they're strong arguments in favor of my plans. There is practically nothing a dog enjoys more than marking its own yard with pee and shit. I'd like to be part of that joyful landscape, to still be tangibly connected to the creatures I love, at least for a while. I know that I won't know I'm now part of that landscape, just as I won't know whether Heather gets another dog. But I'm betting she will.

Heather Responds to
"I'm Listening—for Now"

Don's title for this chapter is funny because he *never* listens. Or at least I have to assume that he never listens since he regularly asks me for information that I've already provided for him maybe five or six times. He says he always operates on a need-to-know basis. When he needs to know something, he'll ask, he says. For example, Don's got the sense of direction of a brick. I haven't tried this yet, but one day when he's trying to drive somewhere new, I might just let him wander around Reno until he realizes he has a need to know and asks for directions that I could have easily given him at the first wrong turn.

The swelling lymph nodes were alarming all right. I considered urging Don to make an emergency appointment with his oncologist, but his next appointment was coming up in just over a week, and the oncologist hadn't warned us that swelling lymph nodes were anything special to worry about other than a sign of the progression of the disease. He had told us that a signal that it was time to enter chemotherapy would be a doubling or tripling of the size of the lymph nodes, but they were already swollen, and not being medical experts we had no idea what their original swollen size was. When Don's oncologist got a look at his nodes, he moved faster than any doctor I've ever seen, including doctors in emergency rooms. It didn't seem that he was panicking; it was rather "Okay, *now* is the time to do something."

As for mixing his ashes with those of Travis, Lyle, Bowie, and whomever else he adds to the list and scattering them all in the backyard, okay, I can do that. But Don's going to have to do some preparatory work on that himself because Bowie's and Travis's cremains are now enclosed in boxes that I have absolutely no idea how to dismantle. And I am not going to take a hammer to them like they were piñatas. Don had better hope that I outlive him because I don't know who would do this for him other than me. Well, I do have a niece who is probably up to it. She teaches middle school science in Texas, so she's probably had to do weirder things in her job. She'd just laugh, roll her eyes, mutter "Dumbass," and do it.

Oh, and I am *not* getting another dog. If there is one thing that Don has taught me, it is to love dogs, but I love them individually, one by one. I loved Sam and Bowie. And I now love Lyle, but I am not a dog lover in general. I am a cat person who comes from a long line of cat people. A dog brings a frenetic, unfocused (if enthusiastic) energy into a house that I am not willing to deal with on my own, kind of like the energy that Don himself brings into the house. So Don and the dog are a perfect fit. I think of both as being permanently on a need-to-know basis.

Notes
1. Hillmen, "Richter's Syndrome"; Jain, "New Developments in Richter Syndrome"; Jain and O'Brien, "Chronic Lymphocytic Leukemia with Deletion 17p."

Welcome to Chemo 101: Any Questions?

October 25

RICHTER'S TRANSFORMATION, occurring in about 5 percent of lymphomas, suggests a median survival time of eight to twelve months; chemotherapy in that case has essentially no positive benefit.[1] My latest lymph node biopsy shows no evidence of Richter's transformation, which lack is the absence of a very, very bad sign. Cancer has at least one benefit, or maybe one more negative side effect, depending on how one feels about Henry James's writing style, which features negatives of negatives sounding positive but less positive than simple positives. I found out about my biopsy by calling my surgeon, whose nurse called me back with the not-bad news.

When I saw my oncologist yesterday, he repeated the double negative and pointed out that the biopsy report of a high ki67 protein level, responsible for cell proliferation, helped to explain my explosively growing nodes. ki67 is at least this: a not-good. It's not known whether it is a bad not-good, meaning that it would have negative prognosis value. We still do not know whether I have the 17p deletion, which so far as anyone can tell is indeed a bad not-good, correlated as it is with rapid proliferation and prognosis of short survival time. As the Lymphoma Research Foundation's 2010 *Understanding CLL/SLL* guide says, "Chromosome 17 carries the p53 gene, which has an effect on regulating cell death (apoptosis). The normal functioning of the p53 gene is important in the response to chemotherapy. Loss of part of chromosome 17 is associated with particularly aggressive CLL."[2] Estimates are that I will receive a copy of the full cytogenetic panel on Thursday this week, the first week of chemotherapy, about one day after my Chemo 101 nurse instructor tells me that I will feel as if I have "hit a wall." I can't imagine what hitting that wall feels like. Does it mean unbearable pain, unimaginable fatigue, feeling unable to go any further? It is undoubtedly a metaphor, but is it a metaphor for a physical symptom or a metaphor for yet another metaphor? All I know now is that it doesn't sound like something you'd wish for on Christmas morning.

If occasionally my oncologist and many of the medical research articles I read sound like Henry James in his late style, when James seemed to think, paradoxically, that clarity hid his essential self, the Chemo 101 nurse, although infinitely kind in intent and in delivery, sounds by contrast to my panicked mind like a Marine boot camp drill instructor, or at least the orientation instructor for the toughest gym membership you will ever have. There is no ambiguity; there are few hedges; if you want to survive, and not everyone will, you had better pay attention.

In contrast to Marine boot camp, lasting roughly three months, chemotherapy for CLL/SLL lasts six months, with one week of treatment followed by three weeks of rest, those three weeks of rest thrown in to cushion the relentless pummeling one's system receives during each week of active treatment. I will learn by experience that at least one of those weeks of rest is the kind of rest one gets when one goes to bed with the flu: that is, hardly any rest at all, just pain and discomfort.

My chemotherapy treatment will consist of fludarabine, cyclophosphamide, and rituximab (FCR). The fludarabine and cyclophosphamide kill rapidly growing cells such as cancer cells, hair follicle cells, fingernail cells, and skin cells in the mouth by interfering with DNA duplication. The rituximab is a monoclonal antibody that targets a protein (CD20) sitting on the surface of B cells (a form of white blood cells), some of which are cancerous, some not.[3]

On day 1 (six to eight hours) of each chemo week, I get all three drugs, on days 2 and 3 (three hours each) only fludarabine and cyclophosphamide, and on day 4 an injection of pegfilgrastim which, surprisingly, encourages my bone marrow to produce more white blood cells, not the cancerous kind but the neutrophils that fight infection, to counteract the deleterious effects of chemo on the immune system.

The overall nastiness of the chemotherapy drugs is pretty much confirmed in the number and kinds of drugs one must take to combat their side effects, the pegfilgrastim being the most life protective. There are three different kinds of anti-nausea medications (none of which is guaranteed to prevent nausea), one medication during the first treatment to prevent kidney failure caused by the sudden flooding of the blood and kidneys with dead cells, an anti-viral and an antibiotic to combat increased risk of infection, and a numbing cream to ease the pain of being stuck with a needle in the chemo port. Contrary to my expectations, the port does not obviate the necessity of piercing the skin on my chest with a needle three times a week and leaving that needle there for up to eight hours, at least on Mondays. I have the choice to leave the needle in the port for all three days of chemotherapy, but since my dog and cats walk all over me at all hours of the day as if I'm an annoying lumpy blanket that they are constantly trying to smooth out enough for a comfortable nap, and since I normally thrash around for an unpredictable period of time every night until I find a comfortable position to sleep in, my best option seems to be to have the needle removed at the end of each day of chemotherapy and a new one inserted at the beginning of the next day.

Here are some of the more memorable side effects I heard about in Chemo 101 that are common but not absolutely guaranteed: runny nose, fingernail loss, dry skin, mouth sores, hair loss (see "baldness"), eyebrow and eyelash loss (see "scaring children"), diarrhea (see "constipation"), constipation (see "diarrhea"), fever, fatigue, neuropathy, nose bleeds, infection, blood clotting, trouble with concentration, memory changes, and sleep disruption. Gratitude is the one sure path to inner peace. If I escape half of these side effects, I will have a lot to be grateful for. The worst of them for me will turn out to be trouble with concentration, memory changes, and sleep disruption, the three worst possible side effects for continuing to do my job with any kind of efficiency, sleep disruption simply exacerbating difficulties with concentration and memory. Constipation wound up being the most annoying, embarrassing, and difficult to control. It didn't help with concentration either (see the "Afterward" for connections between constipation and concentration). It's hard to think or write lofty or even connected thoughts if lower bowel cramping is your constant companion.

At just about the moment my orientation nurse was explaining the side effect of trouble with concentration, I entered a temporary partial memory blackout. This is exactly why cancer patients are encouraged to bring friends or relatives who will be helping out with care to the orientation session. I brought the two most skilled listeners I know, who also happen to have the best long-term memories for detail I know: Heather and one of our best friends, who is a high-level administrator at our university in charge of setting people straight who otherwise just won't do right. I think most people would be surprised to learn, as I was when I landed a job in a university, just how many people there are in any institution who just won't do right. In any case, these two women, both of whom I love, are almost always on the right side of the law, which they can usually quote to you, with footnotes.

I had not completely tuned out. I was just temporarily stunned by the number and severity of side effects of the drugs I was inviting into my blood in order to save my life. This part woke me up: "There is a detailed section of your handbook on sexual activity. Do you have any questions about sex?" the orientation nurse asked, as if she were asking whether I had any questions about constipation or sleep disorders.

"No," all three of us said quickly and without elaboration. Personally, I feared a surreal repeat of my dermatological appointment once matters turned to the penis and scrotal area. There was a long silence as "no" echoed in the large room.

Nevertheless, I was curious. Later I read the "sex" section of the book *Chemotherapy and You* (National Cancer Institute). There are partially overlapping problems for both men and women who are in chemotherapy. Two of the understandably overlapping problems are "being too tired to have sex or not being interested in having sex" and "feeling too worried, stressed, or depressed to have sex." I could have saved the NIH some money with a bit of editing there. Plus the writers left out the most important cause of loss of interest in sex: being too damn *sick* to want to have sex. Come on, people. Who's got their funk on when they have the worst flu symptoms in their lives? The most interesting side effect for men, I found, is "not being able to reach climax."[4] The reason this is an interesting, although relatively predictable, side effect for men is that it is *not* listed for women. If I had already known this detail about *Chemotherapy and You* at my orientation session, I would have had at least one interesting question.

After orientation, the nurse gave the three of us a tour of the infusion room and introduced us to one of the infusion room nurses. I wouldn't want to have to give that orientation, with all the potentially negative news about side effects, especially the nausea and fatigue. I know that the nurse, like a Marine drill instructor, is there to help save lives. And unlike how I imagine a Marine barracks to be outfitted and supplied, the infusion room has a lowered art deco ceiling, and folks (probably current or former patients) have donated not only candies and cookies and chips and bottled water for the patients but blankets and also wigs of every imaginable color of human hair.

Probably because it was late on a Friday afternoon, there was only one patient in the infusion room, sitting with a friend or relative. The patient, thin but not especially frail looking, was wearing a bathrobe and had a simple scarf wrapped around her head. When I made eye contact with her, she smiled as if welcoming me to the neighborhood. If I see her again, I'm sure I'll have lots of questions.

Heather Responds to
"Welcome to Chemo 101: Any Questions?"

I knew immediately when Don tuned out. I always know when he tunes out. He stops taking notes and just stares at the person talking, sometimes nodding as if in agreement, probably really nodding as part of the discourse script of what a regular conversation is supposed to look like. There was simply no pause in the overwhelming onslaught of detailed information: the drugs, the side effects, the schedules, the staff. I am used to juggling six points of view in meetings of university department chairs and other administrators and dealing with lots of details, but I had a hard time keeping up with the amount and pace of information. The friend who went with us and I sat down later to compare notes, and we discovered that we had a few conflicting accounts of the cycles of drugs, particularly those that were to combat nausea and what they were intended to do besides combat nausea: the industrial-strength antihistamines and steroids, for example, and the antibiotics and anti-virals and anti-nausea medications that Don had to take at home on a strict schedule. On the one hand Don was capable of understanding this information; he had researched much of it already on the Internet. But he was suffering from fatigue and fear, and that battlefield combination will interfere with anyone's concentration. I felt overwhelmed and scared when we all got back to our house, and these poisons and antidotes weren't even going to be put into my body. But it's my dear husband's life they're trying to save, so I was overwhelmed by all the information and having to stay on top of it all, and the potential number of things that could go wrong.

As it turned out Don got lucky with the side effects in many ways. Sure, all those nasty side effects are possible. But many of those he lists here he didn't actually experience. He had very little nausea, he didn't lose his hair, and his appetite actually improved except for the days when he was suffering from the flu-like symptoms of the pegfilgrastim injection. The worst side effects turned out to be disrupted sleep, fatigue, and chronic constipation caused by some of the drugs he was being treated with, and the bizarre effects of what is colloquially referred to as chemo fog or chemo brain: inability to concentrate and poor memory.

They don't talk about the fear in Chemo 101, but it's always there, along with the pain of seeing someone you love suffer. At least once I saw Don crying in despair, during the second week after the first course of treatment. Fatigue and the prospect of months of ever-waning energy have got to be demoralizing. Then there is the uncertainty about whether enduring this pain is going to pay off with a remission or if it does how long that remission might last. The uncertainty was especially disturbing in the weeks before the treatment began when we were simply trying to absorb as much information as we could, because we knew that once the process was under way Don would be even less likely to be able to take in and understand important information about his treatment. There may be people out there who have to go through chemotherapy alone, whether through choice or necessity. I fear for those people and feel for them because I cannot imagine keeping up with all of the details accurately while experiencing physical and mental fatigue that never fully retreats.

Notes

1. Jain, "New Developments in Richter Syndrome."
2. *Understanding* CLL/SLL (2010), 18.
3. "What Is Chronic Lymphocytic Leukemia?"
4. *Chemotherapy and You.*

Nausea Treatment
(to Be Used Only in the
Event of an Emergency)

October 27

O F ALL THE SIDE EFFECTS of chemotherapy that I feared in that first week, I was most horrified by the possibility of endless nausea. Whether it's from a stomach virus, a flu bug, or even seasickness, at the first sign of nausea, I turn into a limp dishrag even before I make a trip to my vomitorium. There is something intensely unnatural to me about food, some partially digested, traveling the wrong damned way. But it turns out that the preventive measures for nausea in contemporary chemotherapy are miraculous. Not only will I receive two intravenous drugs to combat nausea, I have two prescriptions for tablets to support the fight, one a very strong medicine to be taken every twelve hours starting the first day of a chemotherapy week for two days, the other to be taken when needed to control unpredictable and spontaneous nausea.

The strongest side effects of the chemotherapy, at least during that first week, were extreme mental confusion and, strangely, blurred vision. I attempted to treat both in the first week by streaming idiotic movies from Netflix, those that I knew I didn't need to concentrate on or even stay awake for because (1) I had seen them before, and/or (2) they were too stupid to watch in the first place. A lot of these movies starred Nicholas Cage, whom I haven't seen in anything good since *Leaving Las Vegas*. I didn't watch that movie the first week of chemotherapy because it's a horribly depressing movie and Cage's character spends a fair amount of time on screen vomiting.

On the second day, Heather thought she could trust me alone long enough to run to the grocery store with a friend to gather some needed supplies. My appetite had taken a real hit as well, and nothing sounded palatable by the second day other than home-made pizza or hamburgers, neither of which at that time were on our regular menus at home.

In any case, I was watching an incredibly stupid movie with Christopher Walken in which his character somehow shoots his semiautomatic pistol across his own pilot outside the window of a prop airplane at the pilot of a military jet and actually hits the guy, who crashes his jet. I think, in spite of my chemical fog, that is the single most unbelievable movie scene I've ever watched. It makes me cringe just to think of it. You can find it on YouTube if you want to see it. If you really want to punish yourself, watch the whole movie, titled *McBain*, made in 1991. But I love Christopher Walken and will watch him in absolutely anything.

In the middle of this movie, I felt a totally unexpected bout of nausea creep up on me, but it was coming slowly enough for me to make it to my chemotherapy pill stash to take an anti-emetic. The problem was that all my drugs were so new to me I couldn't remember which ones were meant to combat nausea and which to combat other things, like kidney failure. My notes from orientation were no use because they had the brand names of the anti-emetic drugs while the labels on the bottles listed generic names. It seemed dangerous and a waste of time to just randomly take pills, hoping to get lucky. So I tried to read the smaller print on the labels, which would tell me the pills' intended use. But I discovered that I could not read the labels clearly: I had trouble focusing my eyes, even with reading glasses on, and then my brain couldn't process the information that I could read.

I hadn't the slightest idea what to do. I called Heather, whose phone went to voice mail immediately. What to do? The nausea was getting stronger.

I was on the verge of panic. Then I remembered I had a bit of marijuana a friend had given me "just in case, 'cause you never know" when he found out I was going into chemotherapy. He said that if I needed it and it worked he would give me more. I hadn't smoked marijuana since I was in my twenties, but I was willing to try anything, especially since I had heard and read that lots of cancer patients find that only marijuana is effective in fighting their chemically-induced nausea.

But there was another problem. The small bud of marijuana was locked in a handgun safe along with a pipe my friend had given me, and of course I couldn't remember the combination because hey, it's not every day I need a handgun and because I was experiencing mental confusion. There was a backup, a key for the safe, in case the battery failed on the push button combination mechanism or I forgot the password combination. Not that a handgun is going to be much good for defense anyway since I usually sleep so deeply that it takes a faulty fire alarm battery to wake me in the middle of the night. But a gun would be absolutely useless if I couldn't remember the password to the safe even if the crazed ax murderer were to set fire to our front door to get in and while waiting for the fire alarm to go off, politely rang the doorbell twenty times and yelled, "Hey, open up—I want to murder you in your sleep." So I kept the password simple, but not simple enough for chemo-Don to remember. The key, where was the key? If I were the key, where would I be? I knew the answer to that one: I would be on my key chain. But where was my key chain? I hadn't needed my key chain since at least Sunday because since beginning chemo on Monday I was unsafe at any speed. Where was the last place I saw the key chain? None of these reasonable questions brought even the faintest memory to mind. So I started looking around almost randomly, which took my mind off the increasingly strong nausea. Top drawer of the desk in my office? Lots of keys, but no key for the safe. Key chain in pocket? No way could I get that lucky. Correct, no way. Bedside table drawer next to safe? No, that would be too easy for thieves and nonexistent children too smart for their own good.

Then I remembered that I had a backup to the backup. I had an *extra* key for the gun/marijuana safe that I had hidden somewhere, but where? I checked my office desk drawers. I checked the inside pockets of all of my jackets in the closet (a long shot). Then through the ever-increasing nausea I had a vision, like a movie flashback, of dropping the extra key in the bowl on top of Heather's desk and telling her, "This is the extra key to the gun safe. I have one on my regular key chain, but if you ever need it for any reason here it is. You don't have to use the password to get in." I might have remembered this not merely because of my desperation but also because of the look she gave me that said clearly and with no ambiguity, "You are out of your mind." Correct. First, why would she need a gun? Second, she would probably have immediately forgotten that the key was there. Third, I had already told her the combination, but I'm sure that she had forgotten it (a backup list of combinations was locked inside another gun safe, but that itself demanded a combination and there was no backup key for that one). We should have a sign in our front yard that says, "This house is protected by an idiot. And by the way, have you seen my keys?"

So there it was, right where I had put it maybe a month earlier. I retrieved a pinch of the bud and the pipe and quickly found a match and lit up. Instantaneous relief! I'm here to tell you that at least on that one occasion with that one small sample of that one variety of marijuana, the nausea that was threatening to bend me over a trash can or a toilet any second simply vanished. Gone. Not there. And it didn't come back. And I never had to take an emergency anti-emetic (or marijuana) again for the remaining six months of treatment.

Of course, as with most medication, marijuana has side effects. When Heather and our friend returned, they found me sitting at the dining room table, happy and high, grinning like a child with a box of donuts. I don't know which I was happiest about: that I had found the key, that I had found the marijuana, or that it had worked. Probably all. I know that I was hugely relieved that the nausea had gone away and I was giddy with the knowledge that if the prescribed medicine, which I would soon figure out with Heather's help, failed, I still had a bit of pot, not enough to have a party, even by myself, but enough for a hit once a month to chase away the chemo nausea.

When Heather and our friend walked in, I said, "Wait! Sit down! I have three things I need to tell you!" I held up four fingers of my left hand and pushed them down with the index finger on my right as I enumerated my vital points. "First, I got nauseated while you were gone; second, I couldn't figure out the medication so I was too scared to take anything; third, I remembered that I had a little marijuana just in case something like this happened; and, uh, fourth, I couldn't find the key to the safe but then I did and now everything is okay and I feel *great!*" I laughed joyfully. "But wait. Do you know where my keys are?"

Heather immediately went into a guilt panic: she had left her post and the mental patient had been playing with guns and drugs and she could never leave me again and besides what would the marijuana do to me with all the other meds in my system? She also seemed kind of mad at me.

I spent a fair amount of time calming Heather down, as if she were a panic disorder patient herself, and finally convinced her that (1) I was okay; (2) I was more than okay; (3) the pot was not a permanent solution, but it had put out the fire of nausea this time; (4) I would figure out how to use my prescribed medicines; (5) everything was going to be okay, really it was; and (6) I could be trusted to be on my own in the future; she didn't have to hire an in-home nurse for me.

Because it was only that once and because I didn't know how my oncologist or nurses felt about medical marijuana, we decided we'd keep it among ourselves: Heather, me, and our friend.

I have to say that it was the best marijuana I had ever smoked and if Nevada, that land of unimaginably profitable vices, ever comes to its senses and legalizes pot, I will proudly have a whole closet full of green-leaf T-shirts.[1] Of course I'd still lock my marijuana away with the guns in the gun safe because you never know what nonexistent children or very-much-there animals are likely to get into next.

It took Heather a while to calm down and get over this. She's a perfectionist, and this seemed to her as if she had left a three-year-old at home with a box of matches, a firearm, a sharp knife, and a rabid skunk and said, "Have fun!" when she went out to run a short errand. She had a friend with her, so obviously in retrospect she thought she should have left the friend with me or maybe asked our friend to run to the store for us. But how could she have known? I wasn't sitting there with the matches petting the rabid skunk when she left. She's too hard on herself.

Heather Responds to "Nausea Treatment (to Be Used Only in the Event of an Emergency)"

Idiot! Not him, me. Well, him too, but mostly me here. I felt like an idiot for leaving him alone for even a little while during the first week of treatment. But when I left, he was in bed watching a movie and groaning like a flu victim (and he did have two different anti-emetics and knew where the medicines were). But I hadn't counted on his understandable confusion of generic versus brand names for the anti-emetics since the information was on the flip side of the list of day-by-day dosage instructions.

But let me clarify something. Don's account is a great example of what chemo does to your recall. I didn't actually leave him alone. The friend he thinks went shopping with me came over to stay with him but left the house for a short time to walk Lyle the dog and came back to find Don excitable and stoned. And—full disclosure—I wasn't grocery shopping; I left him to go get a much-needed massage. Guilty! I will never forget coming home and seeing the weird expression on our friend's face: amused, bemused, a little worried. It freaked me out, especially since Don was frantically trying to get me to sit down so he could "explain what happened."

It was a funny story to Don. I didn't see the humor in it until some time later. He says that when he last used marijuana in his twenties it didn't make him euphoric, but this time it did. Who knows? It could have been partially the relief of beating the nausea. He really has the least tolerance for nausea of anyone I know. He always seems to think he's dying. Once when he had a stomach virus that was strong enough to threaten dehydration, I hauled him into our family physician's office. When the nurses and the doctor were through with him, I sent him to the car while I paid the bill. The nurses were cracking up at how he was hunched over, shuffling like an old man out to the car and acting like he was dying. He did projectile-vomit in the examining room after being given an injection of an anti-emetic.

He can be a Marine about some things though. When we have geriatric animals, he's the one who gives all the injections, including the subcutaneous fluids. I don't know if that generally takes a strong stomach, but I can't do it. Subcutaneous fluids have to be given with large-gauge needles that are inserted just beneath the skin of the neck, and the fluid drip has to be right and the animal has to be held and restrained, though the procedure doesn't cause much pain. I can't do it. As you've heard before, I'm not good with needles.

Don once mercy-killed a rabbit that had been hit by a car in front of our house. It was suffering and in pain and obviously too physically damaged to live. About five of us in the neighborhood found the rabbit lying in the street; mortally injured, it screamed and cried, sounding like a human infant in pain. All the rest of us were standing around wringing our hands: what to do, what to do, who will do it and how? If Don had had a gun then, I'm sure he would have shot the rabbit right there in the middle of the suburban street. He did look around and ask, "Does anyone have a gun?" No one did, so he fetched a hatchet. Enough said. So he can handle blood, but not his own nausea.

Notes

1. Among other surprises of November 8, 2016, it's time to go shopping for T-shirts in Nevada.

Through the Fog to Gratitude

October 30

I THINK NEXT TO NAUSEA, I might have feared a loss of appetite most. I entered chemotherapy about twenty pounds below my normal weight. I didn't have much body fat or muscle to spare. Many sources, including my oncologist's office, suggested that food could be unpalatable during chemotherapy, especially with some foods taking on a metallic taste. The only surprising taste I've noticed this first week of chemo is that blackberries seem to have an almost indescribable essence of lead at their center, but that might have always been there for me because until I get to the center of a blackberry, all is sweet tartness. Also, I didn't realize until a couple of months into chemotherapy that the steroids that I received in infusion all three days increase appetite. I ate, as Heather says, "like a horse," starting the first week. Within three months I was back up to my normal weight of 165, in spite of each week after chemo feeling as if I had the flu and pretty much no appetite.

The first week of chemo itself seemed by Tuesday, at least before the nausea hit, as if it were going to be tolerable. Monday started with what seems to be the most potent single drug in the weapons stash—rituximab. Rituximab is my personal chemical hero because it goes specifically after B cells, the source of cancerous cells in leukemias and lymphomas. But rituximab can cause severe allergic reactions on initial treatment in cancer patients, including chest pain, pounding heartbeats, renal toxicity, fever, chills, and a host of lesser side effects.[1] This is why before I even received the rituximab on Monday morning, I was pumped full of Benadryl and dexamethasone, an antihistamine and a steroid that, like a rude slap on the back, introduced me to the chemical fog that begins with the Benadryl and is only now lifting a bit on Sunday morning, almost a week later. One reason that the Monday infusion took eight hours is that the nurses had to stop the rituximab twice for histaminic reactions (racing heart, cold sweat pouring down the back of my neck) and allow my body to recover with a saline drip for a while before restarting the chemo.

Thus far I've had delayed reactions to a good many of the predicted side effects of chemotherapy. I was told to bring a blanket on Monday because I would most likely be cold and perhaps a pillow because I would be sleeping a lot. For all of the first two days and half of the third, I sat with my shoes and socks off, my pants rolled above my knees, and my shirt unbuttoned as far as I could without risking that seventies look, looking for all the world as if I thought myself on the beach in Miami. I was burning up. On the first day the thermostat in one examination room I was in briefly was set on 80 degrees to accommodate the chemotherapy patients who were having the expected reactions to chemotherapy—mostly chills, fatigue, pallor, and nausea. Every other patient in the infusion room had swaddled himself or herself in a blanket from the tips of the toes to the chin, and most wore heavy winter gloves and woolen knit hats. They all looked like very well dressed and comfortable homeless people. Many of them had ear buds plugged in to listen to I don't know what. I will find out soon that in the chemo fog it is possible to fall asleep listening to any music or watching any movie or television program, no matter how interesting or loud.

I, by contrast, looked like the new kid who didn't know how to dress himself. I couldn't sleep because (1) I felt like I was burning alive, and (2) the saline solution used to bridge every new drug kept me rolling my IV contraption to the bathroom every twenty minutes. But one hour into the chemo treatment on Wednesday, I was asleep and shivering under a blanket. On Wednesday I also developed the very fashionable chemo pallor, looking as if I were a heroin addict. I had hit the wall I was warned about, a wall that felt very much real, made of concrete.

The most heartbreaking experience in the infusion room is seeing younger people who clearly have worse cancers than I do or who are farther along the chemo trail than I am. When I asked her, one of my nurses said, "No, we don't treat pediatric patients here. I couldn't bear it." I've seen two women who appear to be in their mid- to early twenties, both in stages of advanced treatment: the pallor, the loss of hair, the obvious extreme weight loss in spite of probably receiving as much steroidal boost as I am. I haven't yet figured out how to reach out to these folks or even to people my age or older, and I don't even know whether I have the moral or personal strength to do so. I don't know whether they would welcome my company, even for a very brief time. Energy is in very short supply and carefully rationed in the infusion room. I tried politely to decline an offered homemade cookie at 9:00 a.m., because as much as I love cookies, even I couldn't imagine cookies on my stomach that early in the morning on chemo. I felt unbearably rude. I can make a very, very good oatmeal cookie— made with olive oil, of all things—so I might arrive bearing gifts next time, trying to remember that not everyone has my food enthusiasms.

A fashion and chemotherapy milestone could perhaps occur in the next week or so: hair loss. Last week I did overhear my Chemo 101 nurse commiserating with a woman who had recently lost her hair. The woman wanted to know, "If they can make these chemotherapy drugs that work, why can't they make one that doesn't take your hair?" The nurse, who had probably heard this lament a thousand times before, reacted with sympathy and empathy that betrayed absolutely no prior experience dealing with anyone experiencing that particular shock to their self-image.

Although I've yet to lose my hair, I'm hoping I do because hair loss is one way that you know the chemotherapy drugs that kill rapidly reproducing cells (like hair cells and cancer cells) are working. Plus I have nothing to be vain about in the hair department. I've been losing it for years. A hair stylist friend has offered to shave my head properly when the time comes. I was shopping online for Rastafarian wigs, but Heather caught me one day and said that it would be a step too far. I now feel embarrassed and ashamed at even thinking for a moment that wearing such a wig in the infusion room would be funny.

I am lucky many times over in this experience. Gratitude has somehow replaced fear in the chemo fog this week. My way through the fog has been cleared by so many kindnesses—from Heather, my family, my friends, acquaintances, and professionals—that it was damned near impossible for me to take a false step this week. The fog has been very thick. I can't even remember that I'm supposed to be remembering most things. I still can't be trusted to drive myself anywhere, which is okay because I get to visit with some wonderful humans who take time to run me places I need to go, like my oncologist's office or the store. I feel like a dementia patient who has escaped from my home sometimes, except I always have a guide through the fog: Heather, my family, my friends, my nurses, or my doctors. They always encourage me, and their slightest actions—perhaps a whisper or just a gentle touch—are for me signposts of thankfulness deserving of immense gratitude.

I am intensely grateful for all the different forms of communication and help that people have used to reach out to me and Heather since the diagnosis itself. We've received more kindnesses than I can possibly repay, although I will try. Resolutions are a welcome effect of the flood of kindnesses.

Clinically, the lymph nodes have shrunk dramatically even during this first week. I'd never thought of it, but all those dead cancerous cells have to go somewhere. They don't just evaporate or get zapped into a different space-time reality. They have to pass through my kidneys and out my body the normal way kidney waste is expelled. That's why I have to take acyclovir twice a day and the Bactrim on weekends, to avoid kidney infections, and why I have to drink eight bottles of water per day, which is a special form of torture. New blood tests are scheduled for Wednesday. Today is Sunday. My oncologist called our house this morning, kindly asked how I was doing, listened carefully, and told me that the latest cytogenetic panel reports no new mutations in the cancer. I feel like the luckiest man in this foggy world. But now I gotta go pee.

Heather Responds to
"Through the Fog to Gratitude"

I couldn't trust him before to do the right thing, like drink enough water. I've been telling him for years that he doesn't drink enough water and that his kidneys are probably like two shriveled-up prunes. I don't use that joke anymore, but I'm constantly nagging him about the water. He still doesn't drink enough water, but he's drinking more, and now it's even harder for him because he feels sick almost all the time during the week of the chemo and the following week as well.

The lymph nodes have visibly shrunk, and that's a relief. He looked terrible before he entered chemo, all pale and swollen in his neck and face. His lymph nodes were so swollen it looked like they were growing on top of one another.

Due to his own frustration with staying on top of his medication schedule, we bought a two-sided pill-scheduling box that holds a full week of medications divided for morning and evening. He doesn't know it, but I check his medications to make sure they are lined out on the pill dispenser properly and at the end of every day I look to see that he's taken them. After that scare last week with the anti-emetic confusion, I'm not going to take any chances.

We've also attached the medication instructions to his bathroom mirror.

There are so many things that can go wrong at this stage, it's hard to worry about everything: mutations, failure to respond to the therapy (which would then have to be changed), Don failing to take his medications on time each day, not drinking enough water. He tells me not to worry, but I worry anyway.

I know that my friends are worried about me as well. One of our best friends took me aside this week and said, "It's not all about Don, you know. You have to take care of yourself too." It's hard to imagine if and when this will all be over, when Don will be in a long remission and we can stop worrying about every little thing all the time. Worrying serves no purpose, as Don learned in therapy years ago, and it's best to stay in the moment. But there are still many things we can do to increase his chances of survival for a number of years.

Notes

1. "Rituxan."

How Are You?
Great, Thanks, and You?

November 8

I SAW MY ONCOLOGIST YESTERDAY, a week out from my first chemotherapy treatment. My white blood cell count is damned near
normal, just a bit high, mainly because the good infection-fighting
neutrophil level is abnormally high, thanks to the pegfilgrastim.
The oxygen- and energy-bearing red blood cell count is normal,
blood clotting platelets are normal—everything is going extraordinarily well. My oncologist palpated the nodes that were so
grotesquely swollen just two weeks ago and pronounced them
normal. I had of course obsessively palpated my nodes in advance
of the appointment and found some bean-like remnants. I pointed
these out to my oncologist, and he said they are quite likely pockets of dead cells, probably not fit for dinnertime conversation but
for all that not life threatening. The lymph nodes in my neck and
above my collar bone and in my groin and armpits all were swollen at least as large as golf balls. They were huge. And now they are
empty except for a few dead cells that haven't yet been flushed out
by my overworked lymphatic system. Overall, it's looking great!

On Thursday of the first week of chemotherapy, I received
my first injection of pegfilgrastim, which I completely forgot to
write about in the last chapter because of chemo fog. The pegfilgrastim ships directly from a specialty pharmacy. Soon to go
generic, the drug encourages rapid neutrophil growth while
simultaneously draining my bank account by about $600 per

month, approximately one-fifth the total cost of each of six treatments with my insurance. If I'm not complaining, and I'm not, it's because I'm lucky enough to be able to afford this monthly hit to my bank account, and I haven't yet determined the potential cost of ibrutinib, likely to be the drug of choice if I fail to enter remission from the combination of fludarabine, cyclophosphamide, and rituximab. Ibrutinib is also the expected choice were I to enter remission and then relapse with CLL/SLL, a likely if highly undesired sequence of events eventually. According to the 2016 edition of the Lymphoma Research Foundation's *Understanding CLL/SLL*, "Ibrutinib (Imbruvica) blocks a tyrosine kinase [a protein] called Bruton tyrosine kinase (BTK). BTK normally helps B cells grow and form blood in tissues, especially the lymph nodes; it also does this in CLL/SLL cells. Consequently, by blocking the function of BTK, ibrutinib helps stop or slow down the growth of CLL/SLL cells."[1]

I was warned repeatedly that the major side effects of the pegfilgrastim, which was administered on Halloween by a kind nurse dressed in what I think was a ninja turtle costume, are flu-like symptoms and perhaps bone pain in the legs. All the nurses that I saw in the hallways were dressed for Halloween as cartoon characters I didn't recognize. I asked my nurse who she was dressed as because I wasn't sure I could reliably identify a ninja turtle. The nurse said she didn't know but thought that it had something to do with turtles; her child made her costume and dressed her, which I thought was a nice turn of events: child dresses Mom for work. And the nurse, who was probably half my age, doesn't understand the cartoons that her child watches. All of this makes me feel old, which paradoxically makes me feel lucky. The nurse gave me the injection just subdermally on the inside of the arm, which sounds far more painful than it was after the first sting. She took the time to slowly and deliberately massage the pegfilgrastim into my arm for a couple of minutes. She didn't have to take the time to do that, but she did. I felt absolutely no pain in my arm from that injection for the remainder of the week. She was my nurse for the blood draw yesterday, and I thanked her for that massage. Naturally she didn't remember it because she probably gives twenty of these injections and massages a week.

"You were dressed as a ninja turtle," I said, to jog her memory.

"Oh, yeah, Halloween."

"You gave me a ninja massage. The injection didn't hurt at all. No pain."

"Must have been the massage."

"Yep. I really appreciate it."

Then she took one of those finger-prick torture devices and sucked up the blood in those tiny little vampire vials for my blood panel. "Can't massage that, sorry."

"No problem."

As I've mentioned before, the pegfilgrastim is necessary to build back up the number of my infection-fighting neutrophils, the ninjas of white blood cells. The side effect from that pegfilgrastim injection, lasting from Thursday through Sunday morning, was mostly a total-body achy flu-like experience, truly the worst part of the whole chemotherapy treatment in my retrospective judgment. The first drug suggested for this fake flu that feels like the real thing is Tylenol, which I don't like to take unless absolutely necessary. It's hard on the liver, as everyone knows. Claritin was also recommended as working for some folks; I took both with no noticeable effect on my symptoms.

I started driving again this week, just two days ago. I'm out of the fog but prone to car sickness now even when driving myself. I ran by the office to pick up a pile of mail, saying hello very briefly from a distance to one friend. Then I went to Whole Foods, again staying as far from people as possible, to score some blackberry-flavored water, which is what I prefer to drink during my forced hydration of 128 fluid ounces of water per day. I'm drinking these eight 16-ounce bottles of water a day now, not only to protect my kidneys against the dead and dying cells in my body, which I've already explained, but also to protect my body against all the chemotherapeutic poisons in my system. I'm predicting that my skin will be indistinguishable from a photoshopped celebrity in *Bon Appétit* in six to ten days. In the meantime I'm discovering what it must be like to be a small woman with a small bladder. When I commented on how frequently I was having to urinate, one of the nurses said that now I knew what it was like to be pregnant. Well, I doubt I have the slightest idea of what it's like to be pregnant, but I did have to ask where the bathrooms were at Whole Foods. I need to decorate my bathroom at home with some interesting art or something since I spend a significant portion of my time standing in there, staring at the wall. I'm up about every hour and a half during the night.

I wake up a lot earlier these days than I used to, and I'm always hungry when I wake up. Having breakfast with Heather every morning has been really enjoyable, although it has cut in on her normally peaceful morning reading time. Two mornings ago I loudly gave thanks "at least for the ability to pee standing up." Heather said something that would sound ungracious if I repeated it here, but the sentence ended with the phrase "especially when I'm out on a damned boat." One thing I'm learning in expressing all this gratitude every day is that you have to be careful to whom you express your gratitude and how you express it. I doubt that charity and gratitude can or even should be practiced solely in private; but even I know not to publicly announce my dramatically falling WBC in my next chemo treatment.

Sitting around all day at home alone reading and writing while recovering from chemo is hard on my social skills, which are not my best trait to begin with. In preparation for meeting with my onc this week, I had to have blood drawn at a local lab two days ago. So after the short run for mail and the shopping expedition to Whole Foods, which I extended for an hour to pick up ingredients for homemade pizza and just tour the wonder that is Whole Foods, I drove to my usual lab on the other side of town. I'd always gotten lucky before, but this time the waiting room was crowded—even overcrowded. A doctor was cluelessly blocking the door, preventing a man in a wheelchair from getting through to have his blood drawn. The man became more and more visibly agitated as the lab technician kept calling his name and the doctor went on talking loudly and obliviously on his cell phone about wanting this or that test ordered for a certain patient. Which is at least one reason why cell phone usage is banned in most waiting rooms. Who knows how many HIPAA (Health Insurance Portability and Accountability Act) laws that physician broke in his time looming in the doorway? Even at the university most of us know that it is extremely bad form to talk about a colleague's medical problems to anyone but that colleague and only if that colleague is a friend and brings it up first.

It took two patients sitting nearby tugging on the doctor's shirt and pointing to get him to realize that he was blocking the door. When I signed in, I said in as sympathetic a voice as I could muster, "You guys are kind of busy today, huh?" I knew I was in trouble when the receptionist said in an argumentative tone, "It is always like this." I said nothing, but it is decidedly not always like this. Otherwise I would have found a new lab by now. I made my way to the corner least occupied and tried to breathe shallowly through my nose because there were patients wheezing and sneezing left, right, and middle.

Forty minutes later I was called back by a lab technician to have blood drawn. I greeted her, but she just vaguely raised an arm in the direction of the cubicle that I was to wait in while she drew blood from two patients still ahead of me. When she did arrive ten minutes later, I was dehydrated (it showed in the blood test results) and more than a little tired. We made eye contact. I smiled; she responded with nothing, a stone face looking at yet another of her tired and irritable patients for the day. She did halfheartedly ask how I was, and I halfheartedly shrugged as if to say, "Not that well," clearly a social misstep. I knew that immediately. In that misstep, I then realized that I had overextended myself that day by trying to run too many errands on my first day out. I was at that moment also hoping it was possible to express a bit of weariness to someone who is after all part of the healthcare system. But she replied, "Just another day in paradise, eh?" with that same blank I-hate-my-patients look, as if I hadn't a thing to complain about. I replied, "Yes." I could have said, "No, I have leukemia and this is the first day I've gotten out of the house after my first week of chemotherapy." But not everybody gives a shit that I have cancer, and this woman clearly belonged in that group. We said nothing to one another during the remainder of the procedure.

In the midst of cancer treatment, my normal first-world problems come and go. Somehow in the last two days I chipped a front tooth. I do not know how this is possible, since it is only slight exaggeration to record that 80 percent of my diet is ice cream, frozen yogurt, and sorbet and the other 20 percent vegetarian pizza. I love my dentists and their assistants. Each year they donate an entire business day's worth of free dentistry to homeless people in our city. I donated money this year toward this cause, not because it helped out with the cost in any significant way but because I think my dentists, their assistants, and their staff might like knowing that their patients who are lucky enough to afford treatment appreciate what they are doing for the less fortunate. During the repair today, my dental hygienist popped in to say hello and ask about the progress of the chemotherapy. She was kind enough to say that she had just recently been thinking of me and wondering how I was doing. I said, "Great, thanks, and you?" And I meant every damn word!

Heather Responds to
"How Are You? Great, Thanks, and You?"

The change in Don's appearance is startling. I don't think either one of us realized just how distorted his face and neck had become since the onset of the swelling of the lymph nodes. He slept most of the pegfilgrastim flu away, so I didn't really notice the change until the chemo pallor disappeared and he emerged from his man cave. We're sleeping in separate bedrooms since he's up so frequently during the night. He was waking me up constantly. And this way I don't wake him up unnecessarily in the morning, especially while he's recovering from the chemo flu. The dramatic change in his appearance is encouraging, I think to both of us, since we have five more treatments to go through and have been warned that the side effects of the chemo get worse with each treatment.

I told him to make an appointment online in order to avoid having to wait at the lab, but this is just one of the many things I realize that I'll have to repeat until he does it because he remembers nothing. It's almost as if he is in a permanent alcoholic blackout. Nothing sticks. So I've started writing down practically everything, including when I'll be home in the afternoon or evening so that he doesn't have to call me when I'm at the gym or having a massage, for instance.

As for his encounter with the unpleasant lab technician, he broods on such encounters, wondering what he did wrong. It happens sometimes, I tell him. The last time I ran across a random asshole, I was walking our last dog, Bowie, by myself because Don was too sick with the real flu to go. I decided to walk the ditch trail, which starts in a local park about a block from our house. There are signs posted everywhere that dogs must be on leash, but it is rare to see a dog, other than our own, on leash there, although some of the more responsible owners at least carry one to put on when encountering another dog. Bowie and I were walking the trail unmolested until a pony-tailed woman and three big dogs off leash started heading straight for us. I pulled Bowie to the side of the trail to avoid contact, but the dogs ran right up to Bowie, who growled at the threat. The first thing the woman says to me, the very first thing, is "That's a problem. Dogs are more aggressive when they are on leash. You shouldn't walk your dog on leash." I said, "The law is that *all* dogs should be on leash." She said, "You shouldn't be walking that dog on this trail. Your dog is obnoxious, and you are an asshole." She called her dogs down the trail away from us. The damned thing is that once when both Don and I were walking the ditch trail with Bowie, I remember Don and this same pony-tailed woman chatting it up. Her dogs were well behaved that day and didn't bother Bowie. So I came home and told Don about his "girlfriend and her dogs" giving me and Bowie a hard time. Then I called the police and animal control. A total waste of time. So I never walk the ditch trail with Lyle because I don't want to deal with loose dogs and their awful owners. Don is always startled by my assertiveness in dealing with assholes. I wouldn't have given his cranky phlebotomist a second thought.

Notes

1. *Understanding* CLL/SLL *(2016), 63.*

Back So Soon?

THREE WEEKS OUT from the first of my six chemo treatments, I still have most of the hair I started chemo with. I'm beginning to understand the purpose of each of the ten medications I take per day. I'm also feeling better than I've felt in at least two years. I have been overwhelmed by kindnesses from people I know and some I didn't know until they stepped forward to help. Some conditions I had before chemo are coming back, but my blood counts are still good, although my onc didn't show me the last results (I think probably because he was really busy the morning I saw him; I trust him in all things). I already like him. What's not to like? He's really friendly, he's detailed, he seems to care deeply about how well I'm doing. Anyway, he says my counts were good, as of last Friday.

The rashes, the extreme itching (which makes it hard to sleep or appear in public without attracting suspicious stares because of the irresistible scratching), and the acne have returned, although the acne is only on the right side of my face now. I have lesions in a cluster of three on my right cheek, one on the right side of the tip of my nose, and two on the balding crown of my head on the right side. I have one lump the size of a pomegranate seed just to the right side of my right eye, and a suspicious protruding larger lump where the most alarming swollen lymph node was located. My onc zeroed in on that lump first thing on Friday. He said, "What's that?" I replied, "My second adolescence, I think." He

131

palpated it to be sure and shrugged, which I took to be a good sign. I would google "lateralized pustules, CLL, SLL" but I'm beginning to get a pretty good idea of what's on the Web and what's not about CLL/SLL.

Until the rashes, the itching, and the acne returned, I had pronounced myself, silently and unconsciously and delusionally, to be in remission. It was wonderful for a week after I had emerged from the chemo fog and the faux flu. My skin had cleared up. I hadn't noticed it happening because in the fog, you really can't see two feet in front of your face and even then it's hard to recognize whatever is that close. I estimate that my face had shrunk in grotesque lumpiness by at least a third. I looked like myself again. I had a neck again instead of just a misshapen trunk of swollen lymph nodes starting under my chin and both ears and extending down into and under my collarbone. I enjoyed looking at my face again, no small accomplishment for someone whose closest doppelgängers in the movies, as I've said, are alternately Don Knotts and Christopher Walken (in his SNL role as the Sophisticate). I've also been compared to Buford Pusser, but that was only when I was (legally) packing a Beretta 9mm to the slightly shady far east end of Fourth St. for my faculty profile photo shoot.

Now I'm back to pasting my face with benzoyl peroxide in hopes of shrinking the bumps, so I look kind of like a self-conscious balding thirteen-year-old with bad acne but only on one side of his face. I estimate I spent two days feeling sorry for myself when these symptoms returned, but Heather's repetition of "That's why they treat you for six months" finally made it through the brain barrier, and I am looking forward to kicking this bullying bastard while it's down. Kick its fucking teeth in. No mercy, none. I could enter the second round as early as Monday, depending on what my blood values reveal on Monday, or whether the nodes reassert themselves aggressively. I've found several nodes by obsessively palpating. I point these out again to my oncologist; he feels them and warns, not for the first time, that he honestly can't tell yet whether they are swelling again or whether these are just pockets of dead cells that haven't yet cleared out of my system. (I found out three months later that he was worried they were swelling again but wasn't telling me.) The second interpretation makes sense to me because they are tender on palpation, something the proudly swollen cancerous nodes weren't. Oddly, cancerous lymph nodes are not painful until they get so big that they begin pressing on surrounding nerves. You can obsessively mash on them all day long and it doesn't hurt, all the while doing absolutely no good or harm, so far as I know, although it's probably not a good idea to annoy them too much.

I continue to wake early and disturb Heather's normally quiet breakfast time reading with the cats. But I think she's secretly happy to eat breakfast with me. She's also at her funniest in the morning. Two days ago she said something so funny (I'm disappointed in myself for not having my notebook with me to write it down) that it made me shoot water out my nose. She told me tonight at dinner in response to some minor forgetfulness on my part, "I can't *always* be covering your ass," which also would have caused water to shoot out my nose if I'd been drinking any. Thankfully I had just swallowed. I quickly grabbed a pizza-stained napkin and scribbled the witticism down. I told her that I wasn't entirely comfortable being Boswell to her Johnson since I honestly consider myself the funny one in the house, even though she claims almost daily that no, she is the funny one. She might be right. I can't remember ever making her shoot water or wine out her nose.

I don't miss the symptoms of cancer at all. In fact, once past the side effects of the first round of treatment, I pushed out of my mind that I had five treatments to go, in total six months of treatment and then another six months until full recovery, if things went well. I don't think it would be easy to keep one's spirits up without the protection of some level of denial about how long the treatments will continue, and the fact, which I had somehow missed completely in orientation, that the side effects of the chemo are likely to get worse the longer I remain in treatment. But I'm foolish like that. I used to be the kind of bad patient who stops taking medications the minute symptoms disappear. Same as I still think, idiotically, that once I've had an unpleasant social encounter I'm immune to all other such encounters, as if next time I'll have the perfect comeback perched delicately on the tip of my tongue.

I switched blood laboratories this past week, under advice from multiple friends who collectively know all the labs and all the technicians in town. This time I had to wait again, but not for so long. About ten minutes into the wait, the technician called, "Don?" I wasn't expecting to be called so soon, but I looked around and didn't see any other Dons standing up. I kind of looked at her like, "Me?" but she was busy with paperwork. I stood and lined up behind another patient, but out of my left visual field I saw a man about my age come up. I turned to him and asked, "Are you Don?" my tone meaning to express, "Wow, we've been expecting you and we're really glad you're here!" He said, "Yeah." I laughed and said, "I'm Don too," and moved off to sit down again. As I walked by him, I touched his shoulder like we might be twins separated at birth because honestly, I don't meet that many Dons. I had one in my class this semester, a young guy in his twenties, and we must have spent ten minutes talking one day after class about how rare the name Don is. He goes by Donny, which prompted my fond recollection of my favorite cousin (second, once removed), the only person ever to call me that regularly. I had a wicked crush on her when we were kids. Anyway, as I passed the other lab Don, he growled, "Yeah, but you came in after me," at once indicating that he had completely missed my point about how we ought to be best friends because we're both named Don. I had yet again been flummoxed by human nature. Maybe I'll start signing in at the lab as Donny.

I'm a slow learner, but steady. Next time I'll make an appointment so there will be a minimum of waiting, although this new lab was not at all crowded and I had brought a good book on how U.S. corporations in cahoots with the U.S. government are spying on all of us, primarily through the Internet and e-mail, for both profit and fear. The takeaway lesson of the book (*Dragnet Nation*) is that our privacy is compromised on a daily basis to depths that call into question whether the Fourth Amendment has any meaning at all today.[1] In any case it is a good read, and shock, awe, and outrage are good ways to while away the time in a waiting room.

I was called up shortly after the first Don had had his labs done. The technician was about my age and absolutely lovely. I normally don't look when the technicians stick me, not because I am squeamish at the sight but because seeing the needle go in seems to magnify the claustrophobic insistent pain of a large-gauge needle taking up space in a vein. She said, "Little stick. Sorry," and I felt— nothing. I looked down and the technician had used a tiny-gauge needle with an attached port, in which she inserted the vials to collect the blood.

"Wow," I said, "I've never seen a setup like that."

"Yeah, I've found that it's easier on people who have to have blood drawn frequently."

My veins are beginning to bruise in the arm that I'm supposed to have the blood drawn from. "I didn't feel a thing. Thanks."

"No problem, you have a nice day."

"You too. I really appreciate it!"

The sort of encounter I had with the other Don would have normally festered within me for at least a day or two before I forgot about it. On this occasion, I casually mentioned it to Heather that night at dinner, we both marveled at how frequently human communication goes awry, and I forgot about it, except to wonder and worry about this other Don and hope that he was doing well. I used to be incapable of imagining what could motivate lashing out like that other than stress and worry. An effect of my fight with cancer is that although I'm no quicker on my social feet than I've ever been (in fact, I'm probably slower because the chemo impedes cognition; it takes me longer and more effort to understand almost anything now that I've entered chemotherapy), I'm more likely now to wonder after the fact just what unpleasant visitor has newly appeared in someone else's life. And now I'm more likely to, as Heather recommends, try to send that person "love and light" rather than resentment and bile. I have to admit that I haven't yet really reached the love and light stage, but I have thought several times, and kindly, about the other Don because damn it, I wanted to be friends and now I worry about him.

Heather Responds to "Back So Soon?"

Getting Past the Brain Barrier might be a good title for my memoir of our marriage. I *am* the funny one. The only reason Don thinks he's funny is that somehow his inner standup comedian comes out when he teaches. Apparently he can make everything from syntax to phonology to traditional grammar funny. I can't imagine. I've never seen him teach, but I've read his teaching evaluations, which he used to make me read first because he hates reading them. He'll get ninety-nine out of a hundred students blathering on about how "funny" he is and "awesome," and he'll get one evaluation that is negative, and he'll think about that negative evaluation for a week, going back to it again and again in his mind and talking about it endlessly. Spare me.

He's on medical leave from teaching, and the last thing I would do now is urge him to revisit old teaching evaluations to see whether this new attitude of rolling with the social punches is solid or not. One thing that I do imagine may be a factor here is the chemo fog. He can't concentrate on anything for two minutes straight. It's like living with someone with no short-term memory. I suspect that his obsessive-compulsive behavior and habit of thought will be at least temporarily altered by the chemotherapy. It will be interesting to see how he reacts to unpleasant social encounters once he completes the chemotherapy and the drugs are out of his system. That might not be until October a year from now, according to my calculations, based on what Don's oncologist says about the half-life of the drugs that are being pumped into him for six months.

It is fascinating to consider whether contemplating mortality or simple brain chemistry is the cause of Don's more thoughtful, considered, and slower-to-anger approach to life. Could be both. He was told by a friend of his who had Hodgkin lymphoma when very young to keep a diary because it would help him to remember what was important when he went into remission. She told him that it is too easy to let the small stuff in life play too large a role in one's happiness or well-being once one is through with chemo and in remission.

Writing often, as he does now, might even be partly responsible for the slight changes in his thought habits. To write as much as he is in the middle of chemo, or at least when he feels good enough to write, must be giving him the chance to ruminate in good ways. One thing that has changed is that he does seem to appreciate the humor in life and my humor more than he used to. I'm not sure what to attribute that to, but he's less likely to argue with me now when I say that I'm the funny one.

Notes

1. Angwin, *Dragnet Nation*.

"Revelations" from the Infusion Room

November 26

I'M IN THE MIDDLE of my second chemo treatment. It's Tuesday night, and the fog has settled in. But this time I have a lot to think about, and I'm able to because the discomfort of the effects of chemo are less severe than they were the first time. I'm more comfortable and so can think a bit more clearly and observe a bit more closely, perhaps because the first treatment was so successful at knocking the nodes down to barely noticeable size and absolutely knocking my WBC back to normal. The first chemo treatment week, thus, gave me three weeks of slowly increasing well-being, although I stayed mostly isolated for protection from increased risk of infection.

Last week I saw my oncologist on Monday, and he saw me again early Monday morning this week before starting the second round of treatment. There was a chance that he would want to put the treatment off for one more week, if for no other reason than to allow me to avoid the hassle of receiving chemotherapy during the week of Thanksgiving. He determined by Monday morning that the nodes were again swelling and that I should go ahead as planned with the second round of treatment this week. As like myself as I could possibly be, I heard my onc only up to just about this point and then my panicked brain shut down my ears as I started thinking about swelling lymph nodes sneaking up on me.

As usual I had my superior brain with me as well, Heather, who did not stop listening at that point.

Once I was settled into the infusion room with the saline drip already finished and the Benadryl draping the fog around me like a heavy warm wet blanket, I mumbled something about it being a good thing I was taking the second treatment now because the first had not knocked out the lymphoma completely. Heather, who is used to my not hearing anything after "c" if "d," "e," and "f" scare me senseless, calmly repeated what "my tricky onc," as I now call him, had actually said. Starting with "d," he had explained to both of us, me nodding along but only Heather processing the information, that a remotely possible response to the FCR treatment option was an initial retreat of both the leukemia and the lymphoma in the first week or two after treatment, but then a rapid return of one or both in the third week after treatment, necessitating a quick reassessment of the combination of drugs and a likely switch to a new combination for the next week of treatment. This was a revelation to me in the infusion room, just as it had been to Heather in the examining room. The oncologist had spared me the worry over this possibility the last month, and I had not stumbled over it on the Web. So what he had told us in the examining room and what I was realizing only now, in the fog of Benadryl flowing in the infusion room, was that my chemotherapy treatment is officially working. All this of course raises the possibility of a future relapse, but I'm choosing not to go to that dark place in my mind. And here it is Tuesday night, and all traces of acne are on the quick retreat as well.

Revelations come in many forms, it seems. First, my oncologist is far trickier and far, far smarter both about cancer and human nature than I had imagined. I suspect that a lot of the public, certainly me in the past, think of medical specialists like oncologists as being brilliant technologists, delivering the chemicals of necessary and relatively precise destruction. I never expected my oncologist of his truly delicious depth of humane deception in initially not telling me of the potential for early failure of FCR.

This first revelation, quite naturally, turned my attention to attempting to guess the depths of deception all around me in the multitude of kind, caring nurses who greet me. They check my name and birth date against every drip of chemicals, today saline, Emend and Aloxi (both anti-emetics), Benadryl, Decadron, Pepcid, rituximab, fludarabine, cyclophosphamide, and saline, in that order; monitor and adjust the rate of drip of each chemical; and now, I suspect, engage me in light talk in order to monitor my reaction to the drugs. One of my favorite nurses asked me what I liked to be called on the first day of treatment a month ago. I told her that Don, Donny, Donald, and Sunshine are all acceptable. On Monday she greeted me with "Sunshine! You're back!" I nearly choked on my Tootsie Pop.

At a later checkup, deep in the fog, rambling, I told her that I had always thought about changing my name. She asked to what. I said, "Bond," so I could introduce myself as "Bond, Don Bond." She barely registered my joke, but for the rest of the day, she dryly called me Bon Bon, which I genuinely enjoyed, even though I (clearly outwitted yet again) felt that she was chuckling both with and at me. Now I suspect that in using the moniker she was secretly checking that my reaction was diagnostic for someone not dangerously deep in a chemical fog, especially with the rituximab. I think I passed the test, blushing and smiling appropriately for a patient not clearly completely out of his mind and without direction in the fog.

I am in awe as I write this of the well-practiced skill, care, kindness, and just outright brilliant capacity for necessary deception and sly observation in my oncologist's practice and the oncology infusion room. I realize that I am still in the fog and that won't lift until Sunday morning, several days from now. But the fog last month did not produce any false revelations. It produced no insights at all, nothing but directionless confusion. This month's fog is a hint lighter, still heavily there, but I'm beginning to catch on to the wily ways of my cancer specialists.

This week is Thanksgiving week, meaning that the entire office will be closed on the day that I am supposed to receive my pegfilgrastim injection (the fourth day), the one that helps build my immune system up from the low point that it will be at on Thursday morning after three days of what I think of as the nearly indiscriminate chemical slaughter of my white blood cells.

I offered to inject myself with the pegfilgrastim, which my oncologist politely declined and which Heather violently objected to. The normal procedure, I think, is to arrange with a local hospital for the injection to be given there, which my nurses explained frequently leads to long, frustrated waiting for the patient, especially on a holiday such as Thanksgiving.

The solution: my oncologist insists on meeting Heather and me at his closed office on Thanksgiving Day at noon to give me the injection himself, disrupting his own Thanksgiving celebrations with his family. I am nearly speechless.

Oh, and Heather calmly explained to me today that she didn't inform me of my oncologist's plan to closely monitor the possibility of a relapsed CLL/SLL in response to the FCR treatment. She insists that I heard that in the oncologist's examining room myself and that we didn't talk about it in the infusion room, which false memory I proudly count as my first fog within a fog.

Heather Responds to
"'Revelations' from the Infusion Room"

You see what I'm dealing with here. This time he heard correctly but didn't remember where he heard it or who told it to him. In this case what we have is an accidental coincidence of truths colliding in the chemical bath that his mind floats in these days, and maybe will for the next four months. Yikes! The fog is real. But Don can be at his best in some kind of fog. He often has his mind on something other than the present moment of reality, let's say.

Now, with this additional layer of fog hovering, there is not much that I can trust him to remember correctly, which is why I've taken to leaving him notes for the day: when I'll be home, reminders about the pets' care, reminders about his own medications. I know there are no scales for balancing human suffering, but it seems that we both ought to be spared the tragedy of Alzheimer's after going through this experience. I'm guessing what we are experiencing is only a small taste of the horrors of Alzheimer's.

I know I sound like I'm complaining here, and I can only try to imagine how confusing this all must be for Don. He normally has the ability to concentrate on the task at hand, even if that focus can come at the cost of distraction from every other task. Normally, if I go to his study at home to tell him something, I've learned to pause for a few seconds before I leave because more than half the time he'll ask me to repeat myself; although he thought he was listening, he really wasn't, and by the time he gets around to trying to store the information in long-term memory he's forgotten it because it never made it into short-term memory. He literally has to turn away from his computer or put his book down, look at me, and repeat after me in order to store the information because he's too wrapped up in what he's doing at the time, especially if he is programming.

Writing computer programs, which he does in either Perl or R, is the worst form of oblivion. It is not uncommon for him to fall down the programming hole and not remember to shower for three days, or rather not have time to shower for three days, much less pay attention to me and the animals. He becomes obsessed with solving the problem, whatever that problem is.

One of the things I've worried about, that I've not talked with him about, is what he's going to do for these six months when he literally cannot concentrate like that, concentrate to the point of distraction, because the chemotherapy makes it impossible to focus for long periods of time. He is writing about his experiences now in time blocks of just one or two hours. He may not be able to program during the entire six months.

He tells me that he started this book to combat the anxiety of having cancer. Once it appeared that the chemotherapy was working, I suspect that he kept the writing project up in order to give himself a work goal that he could achieve within the limitations of his attention span.

My Real Selves

December 9

FLANNERY O'CONNOR, WHO FELL ILL with systemic lupus erythematosus at age twenty-five and died from the effects of the disease at thirty-nine, once wrote to a good friend that serious illness before death is a mercy.[1] I suspect that I would have felt perfectly blessed if I had continued my practically carefree way into my eighties or nineties, fell ill from pneumonia for two days, just long enough to think about it, and then died. I think sometimes that I do understand why she wrote that and she probably felt deeply that her lupus was a gift of sorts. Serious illness frequently and stereotypically remakes what we understand to be the self into a more thoughtful, more spiritual, more fill-in-the-blank kind of self. But that self is as mutable and unpredictable as Walt Whitman's self-contradictory "multitudes." O'Connor suffered for more than thirteen years from the effects of the lupus and the side effects of the treatment for the lupus, both of which sound very much like some of the effects of CLL/SLL and the side effects of the chemotherapy for it: hair loss, high fevers, rashes, sweats, fatigue, flu-like symptoms, mental overstimulation, mental fog. Many of the symptoms of lupus and side effects from treatment, such as painful arthritis, osteonecrosis, and kidney failure, as well as the treatment of these symptoms by such means as blood transfusions and surgery, are far worse than anything I have suffered in chemotherapy.[2] O'Connor wrote in 1956 that "sickness before death" is a mercy, over five years after her diagnosis. I have to suffer chemotherapy for only six months, if I am lucky. I may well change my mind about the "blessings" of cancer after a few years. Impossible to tell this early.

I suspect the normal way to refer to one's own self in the context of other humans is the self and the Other(s). I prefer to think of it as the self and the selves since all those others scurrying around are as self-like as my self. I've always thought of myself as the funny one in my house. But Heather has been claiming for at least five years now that she holds that position. She used to be, or at least I thought she was, as consistently and irritatingly logical as Mr. Spock. Now she's taken to witty conversations/arguments, as for example in the following, in which we attempt to solve the problem of my next chemotherapy inconveniently falling during the week of Christmas. That means that Christmas Day (like Thanksgiving) falls on a Thursday, the day I must have my "flu"-inducing pegfilgrastim injection. My oncologist's office is closed on Christmas Day, of course, and my oncologist is traveling that week; otherwise I'm sure he would have insisted on coming into the office and giving it to me himself, as he did on Thanksgiving.

> HEATHER: No, you certainly may not inject yourself with the pegfilgrastim.
>
> ME: Why not? Have you ever seen me faint? I'm a Marine!
>
> HEATHER: You will have just finished your third day of chemo on Christmas Eve. Are you telling me that you are going to be compos mentis Christmas Day when every other day after chemo you've been in an impenetrable fog, practically out wandering in traffic in your bathrobe?
>
> ME: Now, is that entirely fair?
>
> HEATHER: Do I annoy you? Very well, then I annoy you. That's from Whitman or somebody.

Heather's appropriation of Whitman's "Do I contradict myself? / Very well then I contradict myself" is exactly the kind of thing she regularly says these days, the kind of thing she claims that she's always said.[3]

The triggers for the appearances of Whitman's self-contradictions, or simply our alternative selves, are varied, probably most stereotypically aging and drugs, recreational or not. Invariably when someone takes a photo of me and then I see it, at least since I turned fifty, I think, "Oh, Lord, who *is* this old guy?" Somehow that thought doesn't occur to me when I look at myself in a mirror. But if I stumble across the photo after putting it aside for two or three years, when I look at it, I say, "Who *is* this handsome young man?" And then I usually lament that I didn't at the time appreciate my youth staring at me from the photo.

When I think of mind-altering drugs, I have never thought, "Steroids! Oh, *hell,* yeah!" But for the three days of FCR chemo, I am also given intravenous boosters of a steroid (Decadron). I think the main intended purposes of the steroid are to enhance the effect of the Benadryl, the antihistamine meant to prevent any number of unpleasant reactions to the primary chemical toxins and to increase or maintain my appetite for food, practically any kind of food. The steroid acts like an antihistamine to suppress immune responses. The steroid kicked in like rocket fuel last Tuesday evening, the second day of chemo. A close friend came to walk Lyle, our cocker spaniel, because I was still feeling too sick and Heather had an event to attend that afternoon. After chemo I slept most of the afternoon, but when I heard our friend return with Lyle from their walk, I staggered out of bed. I went into hyper-drive, cooking two different pizzas, thawing and serving at least three different tapas-type dishes, and uncorking the wine, all just in time for Heather to walk in the back door. Our friend had observed my frenzied preparations with what she later described as something between alarm and amusement. I served the meal to them speaking French. Then I went back to bed and crashed like a skydiver whose parachute has failed. The Lymphoma Research Foundation's 2016 *Understanding CLL/SLL* has this to say about steroids used in treatment: "Patients are advised to alert family and friends that personality changes may occur. Patients should avoid making hasty decisions."[4]

Never having been a serious weight lifter or seven-time Tour de France winner, I had no idea about the mental effect of steroids. And at that time I hadn't read *Understanding CLL/SLL*. Somehow those effects evaded my notice last month, except for some sleeplessness. Now I'm thinking seriously about getting ripped. I already have a bizarre little swelling from my port at the top of my right pectoral muscle, as if I have a gnarly mini-pec that I've been obsessively working on in the gym.

Heather and our friend were still talking about their excitable French waiter four days later to pass the time during the boring UNR/UNLV game, made watchable only by breathless updates on the cannon that UNR and UNLV compete for each year. It's either red or blue, depending on who has possession of it currently. I suppose I'm grateful that it's not a handgun. Heather passed the French waiter story on to the oncology staff, to their delight. On Wednesday the nurses offered to give Heather some steroid pills to slip in my coffee. My oncologist offered the same on Thursday. These are probably jokes they use on lots of cancer patients.

So yeah, Heather's officially the funny one in our house now. She's also much more well read than I am—always has been. She read a good portion of what most people think of as great literature before she was twenty. I once asked her how she ever got through *War and Peace*, which I think she read when she was about sixteen. "I skipped the war parts," she said, as if I had somehow missed the day of school on which the obvious was explained.

Maybe fifteen years ago I read *Anna Karenina*, itself a fairly substantial novel. It took me a while to get through it, reading each day for an hour or so sprawled on the couch. One day when I was maybe fifty pages from the end, Heather breezes by:

HEATHER: Oh, you're reading *Anna Karenina!* Is that the one where she throws herself under the train at the end? . . . Or is that the one where she takes arsenic? I can't remember.

ME: Uh, no, Emma Bovary is the one that takes arsenic. I've read *Madame Bovary!*

Honestly, I think I may have already known how Anna did away with herself, but I had forgotten it. Or at least I was trying to read as if I had forgotten it so that the suicide would shock me. This conversation has been a joke between Heather and me for years, she always taking the role of the well-meaning but bumbling literary conversationalist, giving the ending away before I get to it. Heather and I have told the story countless times to countless friends. Heather has never disputed my recollection of the events or the source of the humor.

Just last night Heather and I were talking again about that conversation, privately. Only this time she let me know, with something like a deadpan stare bordering on a smirk, that she knew exactly what she was doing when she spoiled the plot. I looked at her and thought, "Who is this person that I live with?"

Heather Responds to "My Real Selves"

Good question, Don! "I am vast. I contain multitudes!" That's also Whitman. Yeah, I probably read more serious literature as a child than most people. There are some books I perhaps didn't fully understand as a child, like *Catch-22*. But I read them. I'm still a big reader. I probably finish two novels a week. I may contain multitudes, but the self I present to the world is remarkably consistent, which is how I have fooled Don for years and years with the *Anna Karenina* joke. He would have given himself away within two minutes with that little smirk of his. Me, I can maintain a poker face for twenty years, and in those years hear Don tell the story many times to different people. I am a good liar when I need to be. That is one of the traits that makes me a very good administrator, not that I'm saying all administrators must lie. But among the multitudinous versions of reality out there, one must choose a story and stick to it in order to survive as a dean of a college with hundreds of faculty members, each with their own individual versions of reality. Years ago, I remember a fellow department chair praising a dean at another university by saying, "He's a good dean. He doesn't lie to you more than he has to."

Don does cook occasionally and he does sometimes have dinner ready when I come home, but he's not yet reprised his role as the French waiter. Where that came from I'll never know. I don't think Don knows. It was as if one of his selves just popped up to the surface unexpectedly and, really, uninvited by anyone. It was the steroids, of course, something I don't remember being warned about in the orientation. For each treatment week, the steroids gave Don one day of frenetic behavior, although only once did it reach the dramatic height of the French waiter. The steroids did consistently make it very difficult for him to sleep during the week of chemo. He would stay up until one in the morning and then wake up at 6:00 a.m., which for him is very strange. He normally needs nine hours of solid sleep or he's worthless to himself and others. The reason the nurses offered more steroids, by the way, was so he could "clean the house."

The other side effect of the steroids was to increase his appetite...a lot. He ate all the time "like a horse," as I frequently said. This behavior was in stark contrast to his eating behavior during the year before the cancer was diagnosed but while the leukemia was nonetheless likely affecting him. Then, for months and months, he ate salads and weird vegetarian enchiladas and occasionally oatmeal cookies and whole cans of nuts. That diet partially explains his weight loss of about twenty pounds over a period of two years. So when the oncologist asked whether he'd had unexplained weight loss, we both said no. But what explains the diet? He said many times that salad and nuts were all that he was hungry for. We still don't know whether that odd diet he was so fond of was a result of the cancer or just another one of Don's random selves popping up.

Notes

1. O'Connor, *Collected Works,* 997.
2. Gooch, *Flannery,* 192-93, 227, 270, 358.
3. Whitman, *Leaves of Grass.*
4. *Understanding CLL/SLL* (2016), 97.

A New Year's Barbeque

January 13

O N THE LAST DAY, December 24, of my third and latest round
of chemo, I brought a tiny Santa hat and an ornament to decorate my infusion stand like a Christmas tree. I perched the Santa
hat atop the "tree" and hung the single Christmas tree ball from
one of the arms of the stand. I'm sure you've seen one of these
wheeled stands in a movie if you haven't pushed one around yourself. I was marginally convinced that I was being very clever, but
it's hard to say because around the third day of chemo you hit the
wall, and by the time the wall is looming into sight, all bets are
off with regards to normal social interaction, as is, not coinciden-
tally, the ability to make steady eye contact. I really do believe that
my eyes were wandering independently of one another by that
time. My nurse who set up my initial treatments that day got a
chuckle out of my cleverness... I think. Anyway, she said I could
keep the decorations on my tree. I had wondered aloud about medical protocol.

It was extraordinarily difficult not to feel sorry for myself
Christmas week, if not bitter. I'm sick of being sick, and at times
I've been angered by the financial and personal cost of cancer. So
I understand, I think, the motivations behind what I estimate to
be about a quarter of Internet cancer information offered by non-
scientists. That information seems to fall into two rough categories: (1) the "I changed to an all-dirt diet and cured myself of
cancer and you'll die a sad death wishing you too had eaten dirt

if you don't buy my self-published book, *Cancer and Dirt*" variety; and (2) the "I know something that the cancer industrial complex doesn't want you to know" variety. I'm not naïve. I know a healthy diet is important. I know there is a pharma-medical-cancer complex, and I know that the CEOs of those companies have the same goal that all other CEOs have—building capital for shareholders, including themselves. One point here is that there are a lot of nonexperts out there offering advice on the Internet, mostly for free, on how to treat cancer without all the interference of the Big Pharma crowd. As weary as I am of the monthly chemical attacks on my body, and as angry as I am at the costs of those attacks, I still tread carefully around the Internet, because there are dark corners of confusion, ignorance, superstition, and false hope. With that said, I've kicked a forty-year-old five-cup-a-day coffee addiction and now am crazy about green tea. I eat almonds all day long; and I am practically a vegetarian now. Although I'm in standard chemotherapy as my first medical treatment, I'll continue with my green tea, almonds, and mostly vegetarian diet as long as I can.

CLL/SLL almost always recurs after the first remission with standard first-line treatment. As the website cancer.org puts it, rather bluntly, "Treatment of CLL is not expected to cure the disease. This means that even if there are no signs of leukemia after treatment (known as a *complete remission*), the leukemia is likely to come back again (recur) at some point."[1] This rather fine semantic point put on the meaning of *complete remission* is both alarming and annoying to me. If you receive remission of your sins, your sins are not forgiven temporarily. They are forgiven, period. Given that the religious sense of *remission* was my only experience with the word before I was diagnosed with cancer, I am dismayed that the word means essentially one thing applied to sins and another applied to disease.

Being a normal impatient American who feels mere inconvenience to be a threat to my pursuit of happiness, I am now impatiently waiting for a cure for cancer. If we can send drones piloted by military people sitting at computers in Nevada to take out "enemies of the state" thousands of miles away, why the hell can't we cure cancer? I realize that this question, at least at first and perhaps even on reflection, sounds like mindless whining. Maybe it is. However, given some pretty suggestive evidence, I have been convinced for several months now that poor research funding and corruption in the pharmaceutical industry are at least partly slowing the progress of cancer research. In 2015, 2 percent of the U.S. federal budget was allocated for science research (that's *all* science research, including medical research), while 16 percent was allocated for defense and international security funding. Merely the interest on our national debt was three times the amount spent on science.[2] I don't pretend to understand American culture or politics to a sufficient degree to make sense of what seems to be grotesque imbalances in our values, at least as they are reflected in the federal budget. The word *values* seems unrelated in any meaningful way to that budget. The Afghanistan war recently officially "ended" (for the United States) after thirteen long years, at a cost of over two thousand lives of soldiers fighting against the Taliban. The *Los Angeles Times* estimates the civilian deaths in 2014 alone at ten thousand. President Obama announced the war's end while vacationing in Hawaii. A day later it was difficult to find any mention of the "end" of the war on the *New York Times* website.[3]

The grotesque imbalance in funding between defense and research is not a matter of relative potential profit, at least to the American taxpayer. The American taxpayer is losing and losing big. The Brown University Watson Institute estimates U.S. spending on "wars in Afghanistan, Pakistan, and Iraq" to be $4.8 trillion. And you can include in the cost of war not just war itself but also accrued interest for war spending added to our national debt. The interest due on the $4.8 trillion figure will be higher than the cost itself: "$7.9 trillion by 2053."[4]

Pharmaceuticals, on the other hand, into whose care I pretty much now entrust my entire life, are wildly profitable. However, profit does not guarantee quality. *The Truth About the Drug Companies* by Marcia Angell, a doctor and former editor of the *New England Journal of Medicine,* reveals that many pharmaceutical companies are awash in fraud of one sort or another—with poor performance in producing truly inventive drugs, overproduction of "me-too" drugs (those that are only marginally different from existing drugs but just different enough on a molecular basis that they can be patented for more years than they should be), barely concealed bribery of physicians to keep patients on patented rather than generic drugs, and more.[5]

Google *pharmaceuticals* and *profit,* and you will discover that nearly the entire Web, from reputable news sources to fly-by-night memoirs like mine, all recognize that Big Pharma = Big Profit. As CBS News puts it, "It may"—I would say *should*—"come as no surprise that the pharmaceutical industry is the most profitable business in the country."[6] That's a news source from 2004. Let's see what the World Health Organization has to say more recently: "The global pharmaceuticals market is worth US$300 billion a year, a figure expected to rise to US$400 billion within three years.... Companies currently spend one-third of all sales revenue on marketing their products—roughly twice what they spend on research and development."[7]

Marketing costs are *twice* the costs of research and development? As a lesbian friend of mine said several years ago in an expression of disgust at the amount and quality of the spam that filled her e-mail folders every day, "No, I do not want a bigger or harder dick!" You will probably recognize the word *Viagra* whether or not you want a bigger or harder dick. But before reading this book, did you know the word *ibrutinib?*

Ibrutinib, the potential breakthrough drug for CLL that I've mentioned before, will cost an estimated $98,400 per year per patient.[8] That's a lot of dollars, I'd guess more than most Americans with CLL make in a year. Ibrutinib, a kinase inhibitor that doesn't cause most of the cytotoxic side effects of current chemotherapy, is promised by some researchers (but not all) to make CLL almost as easy to live with as high blood pressure for some patients. Ibrutinib is not a cure for cancer, but unless your cancer finds a way around the drug—and cancer is famous for doing just that with other drugs—ibrutinib might, just might, allow many CLL/SLL patients to live longer. Ibrutinib is not even close to being approved as a first line of treatment for CLL, but it likely will be eventually. In a recent phase 3 trial (which in part compares a target drug with a competing drug) in which ibrutinib went "head-to-head" with another second-response drug, "at 12 months, the overall survival rate was 90% in the ibrutinib group and 81% in the ofatumumab group."[9]

Pharmacyclics, the company that now owns ibrutinib after buying it from another company that took a huge loss, is headed by CEO Robert W. Duggan, the church of Scientology's biggest donor (see "Afterward" for more recent developments with ibrutinib). Ibrutinib has essentially made Duggan a billionaire. So Duggan is now part of the recently famous 1 percent.[10] There are many people who believe, I'm sure, that there is nothing at all wrong with an individual who very strongly supports a pseudo-science/pseudo-religion controlling the company that owns a drug that might revolutionize treatment for non-Hodgkin lymphoma and leukemia. If you think I'm being a bit unfair in the characterization of Scientology, and maybe I am, please read Lawrence Wright's *Going Clear: Scientology, Hollywood, and the Prison of Belief*.[11] Above all, Wright's book, perhaps unintentionally, reveals what is necessary in the creation of a new religion—minimally, a charismatic leader, a large number of desperately unhappy people, and a structure that funnels money and/or goods to a priestly class. Leviticus tells a similar story, I believe, but maybe I misunderstand that story too.

I read Leviticus closely for the first time about a month ago, immediately after reading Angell's *The Truth About the Drug Companies*. I said to myself, "Ah, Moses and his group got it right!" I was convinced that the story of Moses and his people at Mount

Sinai shows what could happen if really important people, like priests and leaders, foul up massively. If such members of the elite sin, Leviticus tells us, God requires not just the fat, the liver, the kidneys, and the innards of the bull to be sacrificed; he demands a whole bull to be burned as sacrifice to him, the entire animal, which otherwise could contribute to the feeding of a lot of people. I thought to myself, "This, my friends, is what we need today to take care of the 1 percent." I figured that God laid those demands for full sacrifice on the leaders at Mount Sinai because no priest or leader would ever want to ruin a lot of barbeques. Ruin enough barbeques, and you're not a priest or leader anymore. You get yourself fragged in the desert.

Leviticus is notoriously difficult to read, full of arcane and detailed rules for behavior to keep the short-tempered God of an understandably weary group of people happy. But then I reread Leviticus just this week, this time with a calmer mind, not look-ing for divine justice for cancer patients and retribution for Big Pharma. It turns out on closer and more level-headed reading that the sacrifice of the entire animal is required whenever *anyone* sins, elite or not. In fact, the only kind of sacrifice in which people can consume the flesh of an animal is a sacrifice of thanksgiving.

I've also done a little more careful reading on Duggan. Duggan invested in Pharmacyclics originally because one of his sons had died of brain cancer and Pharmacyclics had a promising drug for that, Xcytrin, which an advisory board within the company subsequently decided to abandon. Then, according to *Bloomberg*, Duggan steered the company toward research on B cell cancers, among them CLL/SLL.[12] *Forbes* reports that Richard Miller, Dug-gan's predecessor, was perhaps the primary force behind research on ibrutinib, at least according to a "different account."[13]

Leviticus has a fair account of what it must have been like to experience some aspects of Bronze Age medicine. If you had a skin disease (vaguely translated as "leprous disease" in my *New Oxford*

Annotated Bible), variously manifesting itself as boils, skin or hair discolorations, or itching, you essentially saw a priest who examined you and isolated you for a week or so. If you didn't get better, you had to move outside the camp.[14] One of the early symptoms of CLL/SLL can be intense itching and hives, both of which struck me about four months before I was diagnosed. By my calculations, I would already have died by now on Mount Sinai, either alone or surrounded by leprous and unclean fellow campers.

In my last chemo round, on Christmas Eve, as one of my nurses was hanging bags of chemicals from my sort of clever Christmas infusion tree, she said, "I have a Christmas present for *you* today— it's *chemo!*" That's why this nurse is one of my favorites. She's got a wicked sense of humor and isn't afraid to use it on people who have cancer. Heather said my face lit up like a child until the punch line. Then I laughed like a deranged, unclean patient lost in the desert. When I recovered from hitting the chemo wall and the effects of the pegfilgrastim injection a week later, I was so thankful that I barbequed a Texas-style beef brisket, which I hope produced a pleasing odor for all concerned.

Heather Responds to
"A New Year's Barbeque"

What I actually told Don is that when the nurse said that she had chemo as his Christmas present, his face fell like a crushed child. He thinks he's clever and wickedly funny with his Christmas hat for his infusion tree, but the nurses have seen it all before, I'm sure, and they see him for the easy mark he is. What makes him such a great target for humor is that he's usually trying to have fun too. It's been hard to see him go through chemo fog.

I tell him often—though I'm sure he doesn't believe it—that he's one of the smartest people I've ever known. He is certainly one of the most intellectually curious. His relationship with fundamentalist religion was not the best when he was growing up, especially when he was a teenager. Yet here he is a lifetime later reading the Old Testament and actually enjoying Leviticus. I mean, really, who enjoys Leviticus?

Don is much more matter-of-fact than I am about the eventual failure of his remission. Me, I'm into denial, like during the extreme weight loss that peaked in the year before his diagnosis. Remember that during that time he was constantly saying things like, "I feel like an old man. I feel like an old man" and that I attributed this to his chronic depression. I should have known better. But I was in denial. I just don't think about the eventual failure of the remission because that's my coping strategy. This ability makes me extremely resilient. I try as hard as I can to stay in the now and deal with trouble only when it appears.

I have to cope with the likelihood that Don will die before me. I also choose not to think about this now, or as infrequently as I can manage. If and when it happens, it will be devastating to me. But I'm going to focus on one day at a time. It helps being an outlier on the optimism scale too.

I wouldn't go camping now on a bet. But if I had lived during the Bronze Age and been on Mount Sinai with the rest of those poor people, I would have simply kept plugging through the desert. My mood fluctuations look like a flat line. That is a good thing, given that Don is all over the place. I like it that he's so changeable and unpredictable. We balance each other out. If you averaged our mood fluctuations, the graph might end up looking like a normal person.

Don spent months cursing Duggan and Pharmacyclics. I listened calmly and empathized. But in the end, it is what it is—or, as you will see in the "Afterward," it has become what it is. You are on Mount Sinai with priests who simply watch to see whether you die or not, or you are in twenty-first-century America where many people suspect that corporations own our democracy. Either way, if you find yourself walking though the desert, you just have to make the best of it.

Notes

1. "What Happens After Treatment for Chronic Lymphocytic Leukemia."
2. "Policy Basics: Where Do Our Federal Tax Dollars Go?"
3. Boot, "Rebrand It However You Want, but Afghanistan Is Still at War"; Chozick, "Obama Addresses Afghan War's End on Christmas Visit."
4. "Costs of War: Economic Costs."
5. Angell, *The Truth About the Drug Companies.*
6. Leung, "Prescriptions and Profit."
7. "Pharmaceutical Industry." This page is no longer available on WHO's website, although you may find it quoted on many other websites, and it is available from WaybackMachine Internet Archive. Other sources that quote the WHO page include "Pharmaceuticals"; "What Are the 5-10 Most Interesting Facts About the Pharmaceuticals Industry?"; Pollock, "Strong Words from WHO on Pharma Industry." I have written WHO twice to ask the organization to reload the page. I've received no response.
8. Corner, "Ibrutinib's Breakthrough to Market."
9. "Clinical Trial Phases"; "Phase III Study Strengthens Support of Ibrutinib."
10. "Robert Duggan"; Coffey, "Scientology Donor Becomes a Billionaire with Cancer Drug."
11. Wright, *Going Clear.*
12. Herper, "A Lucky Drug Made Pharmacyclics' Robert Duggan a Billionaire"; Coffey, "Scientology Donor Becomes a Billionaire with Cancer Drug."
13. Shaywitz, "The Wild Story Behind a Promising Experimental Cancer Drug."
14. *The New Oxford Annotated Bible.*

This Is Not What I Had Planned

January 31

I READ RANDY PAUSCH'S *Last Lecture* today.[1] In some parts, especially some of the shorter chapters toward the end, it reads as if it were written in a hurry. And I'm sure it was, even though Pausch had a coauthor, Jeffrey Zaslow. It's a humane and very sad story. Young man—in his forties—dies of pancreatic cancer. Small children and wife left behind. Pausch was a successful, brilliant professor of computer science specializing in virtual reality at Carnegie Mellon University. The chemo and surgical treatments for pancreatic cancer described in the book sound absolutely brutal. A somewhat easier-to-take format is Pausch's actual lecture, which you might very well have seen online—easier to take because here Pausch does not talk much at all about his cancer. The book for the most part and the lecture almost entirely are about how to achieve your childhood dreams and how to help other people achieve theirs and in general how to have fun in life, even if you know you're dying. If you haven't seen his lecture, I highly recommend it—it's a hugely valuable (and entertaining) hour and a half.[2] I'm glad I read the book because it makes it more difficult to feel sorry for myself. I honestly don't know whether having cancer makes it easier or harder to read books about cancer or written by or about people with cancer. Yet here I am writing one myself.

I'm now more than halfway through my chemotherapy treatments. I completed the fourth of six rounds two weeks ago, and I was dreading the week more than I ever have before. It was hard for me to believe that I was only halfway through. All the fog and the flu and the pain and the worry and the specialists' appointments—and only half the way there. I never had a real midlife crisis. But now I was feeling a mid-chemo panic. What if it stops working? What if I go through the entire six months and after all that the cancer comes back in two months? I can't go back and start over. My oncologist says that the second response can't be FCR because it's too hard on the bone marrow. I couldn't just stop the chemo two weeks ago, and I can't stop it now. The fifth of six treatment weeks begins a little more than two weeks from today.

I hadn't planned on having cancer at fifty-nine, but to be truthful I haven't really planned in detail much of anything in my life. Heather is a fan of *The Oatmeal,* one of whose cartoons shows a woman pointing out to her male mate that he loads a dishwasher like "an inbred orangutan."[3] Heather's fond of comparing my dishwasher-loading skills to those unfortunate orangutans.

"Okay, that's unfair . . . to orangutans," I said once, appealing to her almost unfailing regard for nonhuman animals.

"All I'm asking is that you practice a little mindfulness when loading the dishwasher," she replied.

When pigs fly.

I *like* living my life the way I load a dishwasher, with no regard most of the time for efficiency or even best outcome. As I've said many times, I got lucky, over and over. It's not that I am incapable of concentrating and planning. I do a perfectly fine job of being mindful when crossing the street on a walk with my dog, for example. I'd never forgive myself if we were hit and he was seriously injured or killed.

A friend once observed that Heather and I are so different in so many ways that it's strange we were attracted to one another in the first place and a mystery that we've been together so long. In our dream states, for the most part, I'm a carefree, perhaps careless, child while Heather is tortured by anxiety-provoking nightmares. Awake, I brood ineffectually like the half-trained philosopher I am while Heather maintains the organized efficiency and purposeful action of a military general.

Among the annoying things about cancer is this: you *must* have a plan, even if it is to refuse treatment. I can't just rely on my usual outstandingly good luck. It's not the treatment I have to plan—that's my onc's job. It's things like how soon do I seriously start putting my affairs in order so that when I die Heather will have less to deal with? I may live another fifteen years, in which case good for me and good for Heather. Or I may die much, much sooner than that, all depending on how lucky I get, yet again. How much of human planning is denial of the inevitable? Magical thinking? If we plan, we'll get to carry out those plans. As if when we run out of plans, we run out of life. I'm already starting to shred old financial documents that I know neither of us will ever need.

There is also the planning that I'm mostly working out in my own mind about how much treatment makes sense in the balance of quality of life. Atul Gawande's *Being Mortal* is a good read to motivate this line of thinking, as well as thinking in general about hospice, palliative care, and the quality over quantity of life, especially if we live into a period of serious illness.[4] I've already thought through the almost certain eventual failure of the FCR remission. Ibrutinib, except for the current economic cost, doesn't sound too horrible, even if treatment does include another few rounds of rituximab, which is the current second line of treatment for some CLL/SLL patients. But a stem cell transplant might be a step too far for me. The intense chemotherapy involved in this procedure, aside from the mortality risk from the treatment, might be a line I'd be unwilling to cross, depending on how old I am and how generally healthy I am. The chemotherapy is so strong that it wipes out one's bone marrow cells entirely before the stem cell transplant is actually performed.[5] For my most recent treatment week, on the first day, a nurse connected the fludarabine after the rituximab and said, "Well, now you're cookin'!" That is exactly what chemotherapy feels like to me, like my brain and innards are being brined from the inside out.

Heather didn't plan on this either. As she said to me yesterday, she married a man three years younger than herself (not sure how calculated that was), we worked hard, we saved our money, we were going to retire and travel, or retire and volunteer at animal shelters, or retire and just go fishing. I don't know, anything but what we found ourselves having to deal with. But we're planning now, with other contingencies primarily on our minds. We recently changed my retirement account over to a plan whereby if the market falls, my beneficiary Heather would be guaranteed the account's highest value after it's locked in. We can't simply plan on my dying before Heather because however likely that may be, there are plans to make that might give me more time (and, as she is fond of saying, she could get hit by a bus). I asked my onc about the likely costs of second-line treatment if the FCR remission (crossed fingers) fails, and he said to buy the best insurance possible because "it won't be cheap." I'm guessing he was thinking of drugs like ibrutinib, although he mentioned no specific drug, because the longer I stay in remission the more likely it is that new drugs will have been developed to treat CLL/SLL.

The results of a blood test today show I'm now in danger of neutropenia, a type of very dangerous low white blood cell count. So my onc has me on extra antibiotics and I think he's likely to ease up on one of the harsher chemicals (fludarabine) in the next round or two. But the worst part of the treatment for me is the pegfilgrastim injection that gives me those flu-like symptoms, not the chemo. I can't skip the pegfilgrastim because it's specifically designed to raise the neutrophil level, what is low in neutropenia. Neutrophils fight infection. If they are too low (neutropenia), you can easily die very quickly of an infection.

FCR is probably the most common first treatment for CLL/SLL, but everybody knows that it is rough on the bone marrow and the immune system. There are arguments among oncologist types about whether there exist patients who are actually cured by FCR. Those lucky few have remissions that have lasted ten years or more.[6] I, of course, am planning to be among the few who get at least ten years out of this treatment. God knows it has cost enough in time, money, worry, and pain.

Heather Responds to
"This Is Not What I Had Planned"

It's not that he can't plan. He can plan plenty for fixing his motor-cycle or truck when they're broken. He can fix just about any-thing. He once fixed the exhaust fan on our stove by replacing an automatic toggle switch that he discovered was broken when he disassembled the entire fan mechanism. The service people we called to fix it had told us we needed to let them replace a $600 electronic control panel. Don ordered the broken toggle switch online for under $10. Rather, the issue is that he doesn't have the mindfulness to plan the things he doesn't care about. So I keep tell-ing him: there are parts of your life you are missing because you are not being mindful about them. "Who gives a shit about miss-ing out on the mindfulness of dishwasher loading?" he asks. There is no talking to him about this. I just come along behind him and turn the sharpest knives handle up so that no one gets stabbed unloading the dishwasher. I take out the frying pan, which takes up half the bottom rack. I move the utensils so that they don't "manspread" across the entire upper rack. When he does some-thing really stupid, like putting in $200 knives with wooden han-dles, he reminds me that he grew up without automatic dishwash-ers. I remind him that dishwashers are not fully automatic. They don't know that they aren't supposed to ruin fine knives.

His motorcycle appears to get most of the attention allocated for detail in his brain. I think he gets a thrill from knowing that if he forgets to check this or that bolt, the whole thing could just fall apart under him while he's doing sixty-five on the interstate over Donner Pass one day. Why someone who has come uncomfortably close to death from cancer and its treatment continues to risk his life riding a motorcycle is beyond me. I was half hoping he would put it up for sale this year. I broached the topic once. Not going to happen. I believe that riding a motorcycle demonstrates a fundamental lack of mindfulness in one sense. "In another sense," he would retort, "riding the motorcycle provides a very intense experience of mindfulness. If you take your mind off keeping the motorcycle upright and in the right lane, you are dead. It's an exercise in staying alive."

I don't know. Maybe it's partly a male/female thing. Maybe he worries about and is mindful only of death and disaster. I'm mindful of everything but. I know that he could die from the return of the cancer, the failure of remission and subsequent failure of further treatment. But I honestly don't think about it much. There are too many other things, more immediate, demanding my constant attention.

Notes

1. Pausch and Zaslow, *The Last Lecture.*
2. Pausch, "Randy Pausch's Last Lecture."
3. Inman, "How to Perfectly Load a Dishwasher."
4. Gawande, *Being Mortal.*
5. "Bone Marrow and Stem Cell Transplant for Chronic Lymphocytic Leukaemia (CLL)."
6. Awan, "Cure for CLL?"; "Is Long-Term Remission with FCR a Cure?"

Existential Dread?

February 10

THESE ARE THE SWEET DAYS, the third and fourth weeks after the most recent treatment. I think it's pretty much obvious now that the side effects of the chemo are getting worse and lasting longer. It took a full two weeks from beginning to end to start feeling human again this last time. So the chemo and the recovery are eating up about half of my sleeping and waking time now. The other half is spent hiding from germs and germy people, especially people who don't believe in getting the flu vaccine, because I can't be sure they believe in washing their hands either. I'll get a complete blood panel done on Monday next week, which will tell my onc whether he ought to perhaps lighten up on the fludarabine, which is apparently still knocking my neutrophils into the danger zone. I wish my neutrophils didn't believe in fludarabine. It's not just the pain and discomfort of the cancer flu that is increasingly annoying. It's the time wasted. For at least two straight days, I have energy for nothing but crawling back into bed after a pee break or a small meal. The next week or so is spent fighting the urge to drown discomfort in unconsciousness. Frequently the body and mind simply have their way and sleep comes on in the middle of reading a book. I've watched the first ten minutes of dozens of movies or documentaries. It was somewhat reassuring to me to read in George Johnson's *Cancer Chronicles*, which in part recounts his wife Nancy's battle with uterine cancer, that the combination of the chemotherapy and the Neulasta (pegfilgrastim) injection laid her low enough in the first round that one night she "felt so weak that she lay on the bathroom rug for a while before returning to bed."[1] On websites and in most books I've read, the fatigue from the combination of cancer and chemotherapy is muted. In real life it can be overwhelming.

Time has suddenly become important to me, more than it ever has before and in different ways. I used to use time obsessively; in college I actually had my days planned in thirty-minute increments, no wasted time at all—or at least that was my intended plan, whether it worked out or not. Now I enjoy time—until I start thinking about it. I'm two-thirds of the way through my six months of fludarabine/cyclophosphamide/rituximab treatment. Another way to think about this is, of course, that I'm four-sixths of the way done. I don't know which sounds or feels better. If I abstract twenty-eight days to a treatment month and measure my life in thirty-minute increments, I'm $5,376/8,064$ of the way through. Although that fraction is ludicrous, sometimes those thirty-minute slots matter, especially when I inexplicably wake up at two or three in the morning and need to read a page to get back to sleep.

I used to occasionally wake up at three in the morning experiencing existential dread. I would wake with the sudden realization that one day (relatively soon) I would no longer exist! *Realization* is really too weak a word to communicate the overwhelming power of the thoughts/feelings of finitude. And how terrifying that seems at three in the morning for some reason, staring out at the darkness. The consciousness that I've experienced for all these decades—just gone. My identity, my self—gone forever. Just nothingness, not even nothingness. Forget about a bang, not even a whimper. Simply not there anymore. In his well-known poem "Aubade," Philip Larkin describes brilliantly the experience of waking up in the middle of the night, reflecting on mortality, and feeling the terror of that finitude.[2] I think the dread was especially common at three in the morning (for Larkin in the poem, it was four) because my defenses were down. During the day it is hard to summon existential dread, what with the daily requirements of making a living and eating meals and walking the dog and paying bills.

When I tell my students about this as a way to illustrate the relevance of Heidegger to our daily lives, most look at me blankly. I've never thought I've done an adequate job teaching Heidegger, even in passing. My best professors in my undergraduate days could make any author whom I hadn't read sound fascinating. Occasionally I get lucky and have a brutally honest student in my class, like the one who said in response to my stories of existential dread and Heidegger, "You are such a sad old man!" Honestly, though, I can't recall whether she said this in response to my story of existential dread or as a reaction to my enthusiasm for formal linguistic syntax, the topic I spend most of my time teaching.

My sleep used to be more interesting than I think it is now for more than one reason. I used to occasionally read the narratives in my dreams. The text would simply scroll before my eyes. And, most annoying to Heather, because she has always been tortured by nightmares, I used to laugh aloud in my sleep, loudly enough to wake Heather from a dream of being chased through a darkened house by a knife-wielding lunatic. The cause of the laughter was never a joke that I had dreamed or a funny narrative. It was always a result of simple, mindless joy, as if I had become the laughing Buddha although I'd skipped all the meditation that should have been necessary to attain that level of sheer, admirably stupid happiness. Luck comes to us in many forms, good and bad, unearned and earned, throughout our lives. I admit my joyful dreams were a kind of cheating, and I understand Heather's annoyance at being woken up by my mindless laughter, especially if she was suffering through one of her nightmares. I think, though, that she woke me as frequently as I woke her. She talks in her sleep quite often. One night my ear was probably within two inches of her mouth when she instantaneously transitioned from silence to screaming, "You son of a bitch, you're fired!" This occurred long before she became a university dean, when such pronouncements, even in sleep, are to be taken seriously.

I've started to read about existential dread. I dusted off a copy of Sartre's *Being and Nothingness* and started slogging through its seven-hundred-plus pages of dense prose. In my opinion as an amateur philosopher, if I take my glasses off and squint, it looks a lot like Heidegger, which I did read, fairly carefully, many years ago, and whose lessons on being, time, and nothingness have stuck with me.

Now I wake at three in the morning and don't have time for existential dread because I have to go pee as a result of having to drink massive amounts of water to keep my kidneys from walking out on me. Heidegger argued in *Being and Time* that being itself is impossible outside of time. This argument is one of the ideas that makes Heidegger so important to existentialism as a philosophical movement. Beings, including ourselves, are inconceivable outside the limitations of time.[3] As a thought experiment, take a moment and imagine what kind of no doubt horrible human being you would be if you were literally immortal, incapable of dying or of aging, say, past the age of sixteen. Now imagine how really much worse (and you thought it couldn't get worse) our cultural products would be, music, movies, books, art. This thought experiment will probably be easier for those of you with children. As for the rest of us, all I have to do is recall that I don't think I ever read an entire book before college and that I once thought that *Easy Rider*, which was released when I was around seventeen, had a revolutionary message.

As if this notion of our selves literally being timed weren't upsetting enough, Heidegger said in *Introduction to Metaphysics* that the most important question in philosophy is why there is something "rather than nothing."[4] That question is not just a question about why the world exists. That question is fundamental to even thinking about the world. He said that it is impossible to contemplate the existence of anything without at the same time imagining its absence, or nothingness. This is why I think, for me, nothingness is normally so horrible to contemplate—because I'm imagining the absence of everything I love in life. But it is not just that. Nothingness is not simply the absence of something, or life. It is the absence of even the possibility of the contemplation of something or even nothing. Horrifying! Hence the 3:00 a.m. night sweats.

Well . . . anyway . . . now that I have a *fatal disease,* nothingness isn't so scary anymore, even when I don't have to pee. I'm not sure why, but it's probably because a version of existential dread has leaked into my waking life, especially in the periods when I'm in the midst of the cancer flu, when nothingness sounds pretty attractive. Especially when I think about how cancer or some other disease I'm not even imagining now will completely take over one day and might torture both body and mind beyond endurance. There are logically possible horrors to think about that are much, much worse than death.

A good friend of mine said she and her husband gave up existential dread when they had children, mostly because no matter how frightening that dread might be, the lack of available time pushes such thoughts to the periphery. Her kids are a daily reminder of her mortality, so who needs to wake herself up unnecessarily at 3:00 a.m. to be reminded of that? She hypothesizes that existential dread tends to lift the closer one comes to becoming intimately acquainted with the signs of mortality. I enthusiastically agree, as the substance of this chapter demonstrates. This is the same friend who came up with the T-shirt slogan "Get the fuck out of my way: I have cancer!"

I have a new idea for our T-shirt line: "Existential dread? Ain't nobody got time for that shit." Oh, and I looked up the "Ain't nobody got time for that" meme on *Urban Dictionary.* As of February 15, 2015, there was a sound file gloss (gone now in 2017) of a young male, his voice dripping with the disdain of the hipper than thou: "Something that if you still say you should kill your-self."[5] Hilarious!

Heather Responds to
"Existential Dread?"

I read Heidegger, probably as a young child (kidding!). It didn't scare me. It doesn't scare me now. I quit reading Sartre after fifty pages. It is true that for some reason I'm tortured, have been all my adult life, by nightmares: the cats being lost or sick and me being powerless to save them, Don being sick and me being powerless (okay, I haven't actually dreamed this, why should I? but it would be typical), and yes, the occasional knife wielder. Don thinks it's because I read horror fiction. Shows you how much he pays atten-tion. I don't read horror fiction anymore. Now I read detective novels, preferably those with hot married sex in them. I tell Don that these novels have hot married sex in them, and he looks at me in a way that reveals why everybody, and I mean everybody, knows that Don has no poker face. His face shows that he is hon-estly shocked that anyone writes novels with hot married sex in them and that anyone reads novels with hot married sex in them. I fear that my husband is a snob in his reading tastes, although he would deny it. Heidegger, indeed!

I promise you, Don's tell for a bluff would be a smirk a mile wide. And then he would be surprised that anybody called his bluff. I *always* know when he's lying. He says that he, like most kids he knew, lied to his parents and got away with it most of the time. I believe it. I think he's gotten horrible at lying the older he's become. Part of it is his anxiety disorder, so that every worry—real or not—shows up as a wrinkle somewhere on his face. Part of it is that he doesn't have much to lie about. He's developed a hyperac-tive conscience (see anxiety disorder), so if anything he is a better Boy Scout now than when he was a Boy Scout.

I don't wake with existential dread, I think for the most part because I believe in reincarnation. I believe we have to keep coming back until we learn the important lessons, like kindness, for example, that we haven't learned yet. I know this world is full of suffering. You can't scare me with nothingness. You can scare me with bad luck or a narcissist human with a hyperactive ego and a sense of entitlement. Actually, I do wake up with dread of possible bad stuff happening: people or pets getting sick, poor financial planning, frivolous lawsuits. There's plenty to worry about without worrying about nothingness.

As afraid as I am of Don dying of cancer, I do hope for his sake that he dies before I do. I think that he would brood about my death, on my nothingness, as he would think of it, and that he would fall into a spiral of regret, imagined neglectfulness or cruelty to me, and torture himself for his remaining days. If he dies before me, I will wonder how and when he is entering this life again. I don't think that it is hubristic of me to think that I know Don has a few life lessons to learn before he gets to cycle out of this physical existence permanently. We all do, unless we're transcendent. Most clearly he has to learn that he is a good, kind person and that the world is a better place with him in it.

Notes

1. Johnson, *The Cancer Chronicles*, 116.
2. Larkin, "Aubade," 1491.
3. Heidegger, *Being and Time*, 39.
4. Heidegger, *An Introduction to Metaphysics*, 1.
5. "Ain't Nobody Got Time for That."

TMI

February 13

OR THE FEW OF YOU who don't already know, TMI is not an acronym for yet another chemotherapy cocktail or blood test. It's the acronym for "too much information," of which many will feel, rather strongly, this chapter contains far too much. So, trigger alert, yet another popular signal for yet another kind of over-sharing: stop reading now if you don't care to read about recent developments in my penis and scrotal areas. That ought to be just about everybody, especially my relatives and close friends, every single one of my students, any of my nurses, and anyone younger than fifty-nine. Get out now, skip to the next chapter, and sleep the sleep of the innocent and nontraumatized. Some things cannot be unseen or unread.

For the one or two morbidly curious medical students still reading, particularly those specializing in urology, I apologize for any anatomical or medical misstatements here. I'm still a bit in shock, as I'm sure you will understand. Two weeks after my most recent chemo treatment, I gradually emerged from the chemo flu. That emergence signals relative normality, which means that most bodily, if not mental, functions return to approximate wellness, including in the penis and scrotal areas.

Well, as you probably know as medical students, men frequently wake up with erections, not that they usually mean much at that time of the morning. So anyway, one sign of a return to relative health after chemotherapy for me is the occasional return of this normally meaningless erection. See, I told you you should have stopped reading. It gets worse. One morning after this fourth round of chemo, I wake up with one of these meaningless things, and I look down because I sleep pants-less and because an erection is not entirely meaningless, to me at least, because it signals a return to relative good health and feeling normal.

But something seems not quite right. I'm as familiar with my penis as I am with the back of my hand, so to speak, the episode at the dermatologist's office notwithstanding. And so I'm looking at this thing and it looks absolutely normal until the last one-fourth, or rather, let's call it the last two-eighths. For the most part it looks as if it is intending to head straight down the road sticking to its own lane, as usual, but in the last two-eighths it looks as if it's faintly signaling a left turn, not a hard left but just a hint of a turn, as if it's intending to just gradually wander off to the left into the opposing lane and then into the guard rail or off the mountain. You'd probably get ticketed by a police officer for weak or ambiguous signaling if you signaled such a left turn.

Heather was already up and about, almost ready to leave for work. I assumed my faintly articulated left turn signal was yet another odd side effect of the chemo, a side effect that I had zoned out on during orientation or perhaps a side effect so rare it isn't mentioned in orientation. Anyway, I forgot about it for a few days until it happened again.

Then, of course, I googled it. If you have ignored my warnings thus far and are still reading, heed this warning: *do not* google "bent penis" or "crooked dick" or any of the other rough synonyms for what Google efficiently informed me is Peyronie's disease. Almost all the resulting websites are illustrated with photographs that you will want to see even less than you want to be reading this chapter. The worst cases of the disease look as if the sufferers are desperately signaling a U-turn, as if they want to go backward in time—maybe not the worst thing when suffering through cancer.

When Heather returned home from work that day, I just didn't know how to bring up the subject. I was looking miserable and stressed, sitting at my computer, with e-mail on the screen rather than any of the half dozen websites I had been reading that day and had rapidly closed when I heard her car pull into the garage.

She said, "Are you still feeling tired from the chemo?"

"Yeah, a little bit, but I've got what is probably more bad news."

"Oh, God, what?" she asked.

"It's nothing horrible, but I need to show you something."

"What?"

"Well, we need to go upstairs to the bedroom."

"What? It's upstairs?"

"No, but I need to show you upstairs."

We walked upstairs and sat on the bed. She looked worried now.

"Well, I don't know how we're going to do this, but to show you I need to have an erection."

"What? You need a what? Now?! Why?"

"Okay, never mind, let me just tell you . . . I probably have what is called Peyronie's disease."

"What the hell is that?"

"It probably should be called 'bent dick' syndrome."

"How did you bend your dick?"

"Let me just show you on the Web."

"Your dick is on the Web?"

"No, let me just show you."

So we walked back down to my office and I showed her the website with the best description and photos.

"Why are you looking at pornography? Look at that! What the fuck!? Who puts pictures like this on the Web?"

"Heather, it's not pornography. This is a medical website. These are cases of a syndrome."

I explained that all the websites described Peyronie's disease as a result of scar tissue forming on top of the spongy tissue of the penis, the tissue that fills with blood during an erection. The scar tissue causes a bend, in my case very slight but noticeable to the experienced eye.

Websites explain that frequently the scar tissue can be a result of an injury that could be decades old but typically results in the syndrome only in middle age. When I was in the fourth grade, a bully who outweighed me by at least a factor of three and who was two grades ahead of me kicked me in the groin with—because this was in Texas—the pointy toe of his right cowboy boot. I bent double and fell to the ground in the boys' bathroom, groaning. For two weeks my penis was swollen to twice its size in exactly the area where the scar tissue apparently has formed. The injury left a permanent discoloration that I haven't really thought about in years. I never told anyone about it, but I did push the bully down a flight of stairs a week later, resulting in a fall that broke his neck, killing him instantly. Or, in that same boys' bathroom a week later, I stuck a knife in his right ventricle and twisted it until blood spurted out, soaking my arm. I barely got washed up in time to make it to my next class, physics, where we were studying lasers. I thought maybe what I probably should have done is blinded him in both eyes with a high-powered laser and then fried his frontal lobe like a crispy chicken leg. So I did that instead, but I made it look like an accident. We had been *repeatedly* warned not to look directly into the laser beam. Or I caught his leg as it swung toward my groin and swiftly sidestepped the intended kick and, using his own considerable momentum, flipped him upside down so he fell facedown in a toilet bowl of boy piss. I held him there until he gradually stopped struggling and drowned.

My oncologist assured me that the bend could not be a result of the chemotherapy. He referred me to a urologist. I was hoping to return to my dermatologist, who already knew my penis and scrotal areas well. When I arrived for my urology appointment, I was lugging my digital Nikon D600, capable of taking pictures with resolutions that rival that of medium-format film cameras. If I had access to a good enough printer, which I do in our university's digital laboratory in the main library, I could make an 8' x 10' photo of my penis—that's an 8-foot by 10-foot photo of my dick. Many websites suggest that urologists sometimes request that patients bring photos. Mine didn't, but I wasn't going to take a chance on the other possibility, which many websites also mentioned, that the urologist would inject my penis with some unspecified medication to cause a clinical erection in the office. Instead of risking the repercussions of printing homemade pornography in the university library, I just took my camera, which is capable of enlargement of a photo on its pathetic and unrepresentatively embarrassingly small screen.

"Nice camera," my urologist said.

"Thanks, and as you can see here," as I enlarged one of fifteen high-resolution color photos of my left-turn signal, "it bends ever so slightly to the left."

"Yeah, I can see that now. That's a result of what we call Peyronie's disease."

"Yeah, I've seen the websites."

My urologist said that mine was a mild case, that usually the disease comes on rapidly and then gets better. He expected my case to resolve itself in time, but he said he wanted me to contact him if it got worse. I said I'd keep an eye on it, which I have, not that I could avoid doing so even if I wanted to. It hasn't gotten worse, but it's still signaling a faint left turn. This is probably one of the reasons why the aphorism "A watched pot never boils" was coined.

I had not been expecting this, but before I left the urologist also insisted on performing a DRE, which is also not a blood test or cancer treatment. It involves dropping my pants and bending over a table while the good doctor palpates, or examines, my prostate with one of his gloved digits inserted in my rectum. More good news. He announces that my prostate is slightly enlarged and that he wants to order a PSA (prostate-specific antigen), the standard but not completely reliable blood serum test for prostate cancer.

You might have guessed it by now. By the time of my next oncology appointment, the results are in, and my PSA is high, high enough that I have a 25 percent chance of having prostate cancer as well. But I probably don't have prostate cancer because high PSA figures can result from a number of things, including constipation and urinary tract infections (see chemotherapy side effects).

The high PSA count was worrisome to me because I naturally and prematurely concluded that CLL/SLL (male) patients bear an increased risk for prostate cancer, as do patients who have undergone chemotherapy. My oncologist later refuted my premature conclusions.

I talked all this over with my oncologist, who referred me back to my urologist because (who knew?) urologists, not oncologists, normally diagnose prostate cancer. My oncologist dug up my most recent PSA test before the abnormal one, from last September. The results were normal. When he found the test results in his file, which I insisted he had, he seemed puzzled and asked himself more than me, I'm guessing, "Why would I have PSA results for you? I don't usually order PSA blood tests." Normally a family physician would have ordered those tests, but my family physician was preoccupied the last time I saw him with the well-placed fear that I had leukemia and/or lymphoma.

Heather reminded me later that it was she who insisted back in September that a PSA test be run along with my other blood tests, "if for nothing else, as a base line."

I've been reading all the lovely details of prostate biopsies online for the last two days, as I wait for my latest new specialist to call me to let me know what the next step might be. TMI!

Heather Responds to "TMI"

There are many things to say about this new development, the most obvious of which is that it is not good to have yet another kind of cancer to worry about. Don is convinced that he's in for another round of chemo after this one ends or at least radiation, if not surgery. I am in full denial mode because that is the only way to stay sane since we don't know anything yet.

I've seen the pictures and the real thing, and he does have a mild case of this syndrome if those pictures on the Web are representative of normal cases. Don struts around with the condition now as if he is a different man, as if I too ought to be excited about it, I think because men find so much of their identity hanging between their legs. Jesus. The dick jokes! A friend who knows called the other day to check up and asked him, "How's it hanging?" I thought Don was going to inhale the telephone in his uncontrolled, snorting laughter. Dicks, I know, are inherently a topic for humor, but men celebrate to excess their inbuilt source of humor. Still, I think even they realize that the standard dick jokes get old, you know: "You ought to get a thumb drive, man. It can hold a gazillion pictures and it's no bigger than your dick" or "His dick is so big the doctor delivering him thought that he was a horse." So to be provided with a "new" dick, one that looks and behaves differently from the old one, must be like a second adolescence. Apparently Peyronie's is pretty common. One of Don's friends, maybe fifteen years older, said that he had Peyronie's for ten years until erectile dysfunction cured it. That one got repeated around the house for about two weeks. You see what I mean here.

In helping to write and edit this book, I have learned things I didn't know, like about the bullying. Don had never told me about that. How do you live with someone for thirty years and not hear that story? There are other things that I did know about. I knew that he was taking pictures of his "left-turn signal" with his big-ass camera, so I wasn't surprised when he told me that he showed the pictures not only to his urologist but also to the urologist's nurse. He said that she asked what brought him in. He said that he thought he had Peyronie's disease and said that he had brought pictures and did she want to see them? She shrugged and said,

"Sure." He said, "Are you sure?" She nodded yes and said, "Yeah, I should probably see them." He said he scrolled through them and was surprised that she didn't act more impressed. (I didn't ask what he expected her to be impressed by.)

For me the funniest part was him dragging me upstairs. What plan, exactly, did he have in mind?

My Afterlife

ONE OF MY VERY SMARTEST STUDENTS said to me once, "All dog books end the same." I'll never forget that bold statement about mortality because although I can't say for sure (I haven't read all dog books), it is nevertheless likely true because that's part of the dog-human contract, unfortunately. Now that I'm in the position of possibly being survived by my current dog love object—Lyle—*and* my wife—Heather—it seems especially important to make the most of our time together and to rethink the plot not just of my life but of my afterlife.

When I think of an afterlife, what I think of most frequently is not heaven or hell or dispersal of my atoms among the stars or even, more likely, among the dirt and rocks in the backyard. I think of all the animals who have befriended me without a word. I think most human souls are far too complicated to reunite with after death, at least immediately. I don't know about you, but I'm not especially anticipating immediate and eternal bliss in the presence of God—after judgment, of course. I feel just now that I would need a long rest from anything that I was created in the image of, or from others who were created in a similar image. Mostly I feel that I would need a break from creatures gifted with language. I love my human friends and relatives now, but really, wouldn't it be nice when we're done with this life to just sit by a river with all the souls of the dogs, cats, hamsters, and other furry friends that we've shared precious time with and simply watch the river and play and nap for, oh, I don't know, a thousand years?

Talk is important to me now. Before cancer barged into our lives, Heather and I used to enjoy eating dinner while watching television. We talked through the show or movie usually, because Heather does that. She talks to the actors, to the directors, to the producers. She asks me questions when she is really puzzled by something. My usual honest response is "I haven't got a clue" because she normally wants to know why humans behave in the odd ways they do, especially in movies. Now we never watch television during dinner. We sit at the dinner table and talk over the day, or she just keeps me company if all I can do is slump over a plate in chemo exhaustion. But we normally talk. I've learned that she has a secret identity; her secret identity name is Tanya. I never get it right. I call her Tonya or Sonya or, even worse when she's in that mood, Heather. I haven't got the fuzziest idea what this is all about, but Tanya shows up every now and then.

Most of my friends are academics, because you make friends with people you spend time with, and university work is a time-consuming occupation—wonderful but time consuming. Just last year I learned something about nicknames from my academic friends. In my bicycle gang of English professors, I wanted to be called Thunder. I was very early on in my own mind designing my own spandex Thunder clothing line. But I learned pretty quickly that you don't get to choose your own nickname. My biker nickname is now firmly established as Twerk, and it has spread to other contexts. It's not the name I chose; it's the name I earned!

Unlike the afterlife, where I suspect language won't be necessary, in this life it's inescapable. And sometimes what you hear can break your heart. Last week, I overheard a friend of a napping patient in chemotherapy say to another friend, "We're considering stopping the chemotherapy and going into hospice because the chemo doesn't seem to be working and it's increasing her suffering too much." She wept as she said this. You can't unhear something like that.

I have a notebook full of random thoughts on language and chemotherapy: "My nurse listed the drugs for the first day last week: 'Decadron, Benadryl, Aloxi, Emend, Pepcid, rituximab, fludarabine, cyclophosphamide. All the eight reindeer.'" The nurses have their jokes that get me every single time: "Now you're on drizzle" for the start of the first saline drip; "Now you're on the rinse cycle" for the start of the final saline drip. I love the macabre humor of the infusion room. Some of us are sufficiently lucky to be healthy enough to laugh in the face of the brutal drugs, the assaults on our well-being, the start of the long slog through the treatment week and the following recovery week. "You're cookin' now!" In a hundred years, I hope cancer patients can look back on standard treatments of today and be thankful that cancer treatment has progressed both in its humaneness and its effectiveness so that laughter can always be about something other than chasing away fear—gallows humor without the noose.

I have only one chemo treatment week left, in the third week of March. I'm going to miss my nurses most of all. Some of them have discovered that I love documentaries on Netflix, and this last time around we swapped favorites. They recommended *Samsara, Tiny, Burt's Bees,* and *I Am.* I recommended *So Much So Fast, The Queen of Versailles, Blackfish* (they'd seen it), and *Honey Badgers: Masters of Mayhem. Samsara* is probably the most visually rapturous documentary I've ever seen; and it has not one syllable of human language. I won't ruin it for you with language.

This past week, I played a game with a nurse who weighs me every single day before the chemo starts.

"Okay, I'm going to guess my weight. If I win, no chemo today!"

"Uh, no, but okay, guess."

"168!"

"Wrong! 170! Chemo for you today, buddy!"

I was wrong every single day. How can one's weight change three days in a row? I even wore the same clothes to try to win. I'm going to miss my nurses.

I think I get my sense of humor from my mother. Of all my family, I love my brother's laugh best, maybe because we laugh at the same things and in the same way and I feel a soul vibration when I hear my laugh in his. Both my sisters and my stepmom probably have the best southern accents in the family. I love their vowels. I love their voices. But my mother, my mother can crack me up. When she read about my left-drifting turn signal, she texted, "It's called broke dick syndrome. Here's some quick fixes. Scream out 'Attention!!!' The other is a condom splint, which is removed before sex. Last, but not recommended, is 'Pound with meat tenderizer mallet and massage to desired straightness.'" As I've mentioned before, my mom was a nurse. I don't even want to know what a condom splint is, and wouldn't you put it on rather than take it off before sex? I've got an image of myself walking around town with a fake boner most days of the week . . . Okay, I googled it, and yes, they're real.

Dad died last February. He was the best storyteller in the family, but he had a laryngectomy for laryngeal cancer a number of years ago. I imagine him decidedly not taking time off to just sit by a river and think. He's gone straight to his mom and his sister in heaven, and I doubt there has been a moment of silence in the last year. His death was hard. He was very tired at the end. I was relieved that his suffering was over when he died.

After the death of my last dog (as an adult, I've only ever had cocker spaniels), I wrote an obituary that I circulated to friends of his. It was an attempt to control grief with language:

After a long (almost fourteen years) and very full and rich life with lots of friends, Bowie died yesterday morning of multiple causes, the most immediate being kidney failure. Bowie held several offices, the most important to me being our dear family member, with unconditional

*love for Heather, me, and a stable of cats—ranging from Gatsby and
Minouche through Travis, Lamar, and Lyndon. He was the mascot for
Northern Illinois University's chapter of Sigma Tau Delta and officiated
as Dog at many picnics, inductions, and pumpkin carvings. He also loved
chasing "bastard red dot" (his laser pointer) up and down the third floor
of Reavis Hall, sliding the last ten feet of each run. He loved walking on
campus at NIU; he loved going into the office and seeing his friends there.
I'm including one of my favorite photos of him on campus; it was a hot
day but he cheerfully posed for me in the commons. Here in Nevada he
loved fetching softballs. Just a couple of years ago, I finally learned how
to hit a softball, in the process of which I learned about repetitive motion
sports injuries. Bowie loved the snow more than almost anything. He
was a really good dog and good soul. I'm sure he's looking after us still.*

I grieved for almost two years before I was ready for another
dog—Lyle. Lyle wouldn't fetch a ball for a steak dinner, but he
loves/hates bastard red dot as much as Bowie did.

Heather and I once took Bowie to an animal communicator,
who also happened to be a licensed veterinarian from one of the
best vet schools in the United States. I'll respect Bowie's right to
privacy; let's just say he was exhibiting behavior that annoyed
his humans. When we entered the doctor's office space, there was
Eastern music playing, a fake waterfall babbling, and the smoke of
incense floating through the sunbeams streaming in the window.
Bowie walked in on leash, immediately turned his back on the vet,
and stared disdainfully out the glass door. Minutes passed with no
discernible rapport developing between the vet and Bowie. The
vet said she'd never before met a dog who simply refused all communication of any sort. In the meantime, I was flat on my back on
the floor enthusing about how relaxed I was and could I talk to her
about my problems at my job? Bowie's behavior problems cleared
up soon after that, as if the threat of a return to the animal communicator's office was too awful to consider. Me, I entered talk
therapy for a few months to work through some job and family

stress. If only my cure were as straightforward as staring out the door.

Lyle sleeps every night curled up next to me like a seal pup. He doesn't get jokes. But I never try to tell him jokes. He would be patient with me if I complained about my day at work, but he wouldn't understand committee work and university rivalries and the occasional sad arrogance of fragile egos any more than I understand, really, my own occasional sad arrogance and fragile ego, whether at work or at home. All of that comes with language. And in the absence of a shared language, Lyle and I are at peace with one another and, when together, with the world.

This book will not end like all dog books because I will finish it before I or Lyle dies. I think this writing is important to me. It gives me peace. But there is a greater peace waiting after the language, down by the river, sitting by the river, with Lyle and Bowie and others who don't come to talk. The time for talking will be done, at least for a while. It will be enough to just rest and be together. Then it will be time to talk and laugh with others, but shyly at first. As we gradually warm up over eternity, there will be plenty of time to choose our words kindly and gently.

Heather Responds to "My Afterlife"

Let me just mention here that for someone who claims to want to sit quietly by a river after death for a thousand years, napping with his dogs and cats, Don sure seems to talk a lot in this life. Look back over this chapter. He's amusing his nurses with guessing his weight, he's swapping documentary titles with them, he's yakking with the animal communicator as if she's there to talk with him rather than Bowie.

Furthermore, I have some bad news for him. There is no afterlife, at least not as he envisions. I think I mentioned I believe in reincarnation. You have to come back to this world over and over again, gradually figuring out what you need to know as a human being until you learn what it is that you are sent here to learn, although there is likely to be a resting period for the soul before incarnating. Don's vision of his afterlife assumes that the Earth School doesn't matter so you just move on to the next life to sit by rivers and enjoy each other's company. Comforting, I suppose, but unlikely, I think.

It's become a commonplace in the press to report on psychological tests that demonstrate how next to impossible it is for humans to change their beliefs even when presented with evidence that directly contradicts those beliefs.[1] I once gave a badly behaving colleague a book on meditation and mindfulness in an attempt to motivate him to change his contrarian ways, at his invitation, because he knew people disliked him. He returned the book to me a month later and asked, "Don't you think, Heather, that we're just born the way we are and that really we can't change? That's just the way we are, isn't it?" That too is a commonly held comforting belief for the morally and intellectually lazy. It is possible to change. It's possible to change entire societies, but it's very difficult. It would be unfortunate if people used results of cognitive science research to justify their own inability to change.

If Don wants an afterlife, he ought to try first to have an alternative existence here, like Tanya. He never remembers that it's my vacation name. If Don wants to be Thunder, I can't imagine why he can't be Thunder. Twerk is not even funny, although Don thinks it is, just like Don Bond.

As for watching television during dinner, I will be relieved when we're back to that, although during chemo Don half watches practically everything worth watching, laid up in his bed of pain and rest. Mostly in these months of chemo Don wants me to tell him about my day at work, which is understandable given that he is stuck here at home with no one to talk to but the animals, even if he does claim that he wants to sit around with them for a thousand years down by the river. Honestly, the last thing I want to do when I get home from work is review the day's work with

Don. I prefer to leave my work problems at work, and furthermore most of those work problems I can't talk about with Don anyway because of confidentiality. My job often consists of dealing with people behaving badly, so if anyone needs a thousand years down by the river sitting quietly with her pets it's me.

Notes

1. Mooney, "The Science of Why We Don't Believe Science"; McRaney, "The Backfire Effect."

My Blind Spots

I'M FEELING PRETTY GOOD. One more week of feeling good and then it's my last treatment week. As much as there is to complain about chemotherapy, and I've done more than my fair share of complaining, I'm fearful of ending treatment because in chemo at least I know that I'm *doing* something about the cancer. There is an odd satisfaction in feeling that I am working hard, very hard, to rid myself of cancer or at least to beat it back for several years. For five months I've sacrificed my sense of well-being for approximately two weeks out of each month. After this next treatment, next week, I will have to say good-bye to most of my nurses, and I won't be seeing my oncologist after the regular post-chemo treatment visit except only about once every three months for a checkup. Once out of treatment, where I feel as if not just me but my cancer is the focus of attention for so many brilliant and motivated health experts, it's cancer's turn to play its cards—and silently. There isn't one thing I can do about it. My oncologist says my blood will be tested every three months until the cancer comes back. Then a biopsy will need to be taken in order to determine whether there are any new mutations in the cancer cells. After my chemotherapy ends this month, I will visit my surgeon to have my port removed from my chest. But with the promise of new biopsies sometime in the future, I know I will see my favorite surgeon yet again. My oncologist is shockingly matter-of-fact about the cancer returning eventually. It is difficult now not to play the "what-if?" or the "if-then" game, spinning into uncontrollable anxiety.

Generalized and specific anxiety hit me so hard last week that I made and kept an urgent appointment to see my therapist, the best psychotherapist I've ever had. I hadn't seen him for five years. Two friends who know his practice had been asking me for six months whether I had seen him yet. I hadn't needed to, but I reassured them that I would as soon as I felt the need. I had no idea what he would say when I told him I had cancer and had been in chemotherapy for the last five months and been doing pretty much okay. But last week I knew it was time to see him again. He is so good that I need to write about the horrible fear that brought me to him before he cures me of it, if he hasn't already. Starting the night after our appointment, I started sleeping a solid eight hours. For at least a week before our appointment, I hadn't been able to sleep for more than four hours at a time without waking up with the night terrors. And my days, all my time, had been occupied with intense anxiety that I hadn't been able to shake off.

Time is one of the more interesting problems of human language and thought. And of all time, the hardest to pin down—if you had such a desire—is the present. The past is easy to see and to talk about. Once a moment becomes the past, you can dredge it up over and over and over again, like a cow chewing its cud. You can even invent things that "happened in the past" that never actually occurred. The future is even mentally richer and more imagined than the past. If you are an unalloyed pessimist, the worst will happen, guaranteed (in your mind). If you are an unalloyed optimist, the best will happen, guaranteed (in your mind). I used to have no idea what this would mean. Now I do. I think I have a heavily alloyed optimism, contaminated by a bully of a pessimist, about my cancer prognosis. I'm going to live another twenty-five years, but I'm going to die within a year.

When I think about the present, the time or place where we are encouraged to live by psychotherapists, for example, I think of it as a blind spot in my narrative; the present is the swirling passageway between the past and the future. The optic nerve must pass through the retina, and since there are no receptors at that place where the nerve passes through, we have a blind spot in each eye, the scotomata. That place, that place right there, seems like the present to me. Although there are experimental novels and short stories written in the present tense, it is damned near impossible to tell a story entirely in the present progressive. Try it:

> I'm taking a walk with Lyle. Lyle is sniffing other dogs' butts when he is approaching them. Lyle is scratching at the dirt and snuffling in the hole that he is making to be smelling whatever is being there. I'm wondering what it is really being like to be being a dog. Lyle is probably never wondering what it is really being like to be being a human.

To me, this sounds a bit like Gertrude Stein on a really bad day.

In language we fall so easily and naturally, if often painfully, into the past or the future. When I was a teenager I was an expert at ignoring the future, or rather the consequences of my behavior. I have a criminal record for climbing the tallest radio tower in the world at the time, right there in Dallas, Texas, in 1972. I was a juvenile, so I was taken to a separate holding facility from my friends, who were older and were taken to the real jail. I was, of course, jealous and embarrassed that I wasn't taken to the real jail. All I told my girlfriend was that I had been "arrested." My climbing friends and I all saw the family across the street from the tower sitting on their front porch. We saw the family see us climb the fence. I suppose none of us imagined that the natural and ultimately responsible thing to do was for somebody in that family to call the police to round up the five teenagers who looked determined to kill their idiot selves. I know I was surprised about halfway up the tower when two squad cars arrived with search lights that found us immediately. The voice of the police officer who told us to "come down from around up there" sounded tired. Once we climbed down, he told us that we should all become policemen so we could do our "own thing" legally. He said he always did exactly what he wanted to, and the best thing was that it was all legal: "No dope, no climbing other people's radio towers, just riding around in fast cars and busting hippie asses like yours."

I said, "Yes, sir" and then thought, "Why didn't I see this coming? Oh, shit, I'm being *arrested*. [Right there. That right there's the present.] Cool!"

I remember that moment, and I remember the fear and joy of that moment of being arrested, finally. I had done so many stupid things, like taking up smoking at the age of ten and then again at age seventeen, climbing the Coors beer sign in Dallas, jumping off the railroad bridge at night 40 feet into the pitch-black water of Lake Grapevine (the rumor was that if you jumped off the wrong side, you'd hit the pillars just beneath the water and *die*), being in the hospital as a teenager with blood poisoning and being so joyful that my friends were visiting me that I jumped up and down and up and down on the bed as if it were a trampoline (when the nurse walked in on my circus performance she shrieked, "Get down from there, you, you have blood clots. You could *kill* yourself, you... don't you have any sense at all!? *Jesus!*"). I had already done so many stupid things that it was only a matter of time before I either died from one of them or got arrested. After that arrest I told myself that my life of crime was over.

It's the future tense that occupies my energies now more than the past, although my mind is occasionally stunned silent by how lucky I am to have lived this long. I've lived long enough that even my memories of early adulthood seem as distant as if they happened in another lifetime. I've taken up, gotten pretty good at, and dropped in turn billiards, tennis, golf, ping-pong, and racquetball. I've had four motorcycles, all of which I've put lots of miles on. The winter that I built my current motorcycle, six years ago, was, I think, the most enjoyable winter I've ever had. I'm a pretty good skier now and hope to get back to the slopes next year. When I was a teenager in the seventies, I was in a generation of young people who "discovered" bicycling. The bikes we rode then, considered state of the art, were tanks compared to what is now available even at the low end of the bicycle market. I hadn't ridden a bicycle for at least thirty years until last year when I bought a Trek road bike that I will never live long enough to be worthy of, no matter how long I live.

When I relapse, and I will, what will I do? What's the next step in treatment? I think I finally understand that there honestly aren't any answers to these questions. My oncologist on more than one occasion has told me that the treatment of cancer in the next ten years will in all likelihood be revolutionized. The person who nailed that realization down for me in the last week was a very kind reader of a draft of this book who sent me a link to a VICE documentary on using viruses (yep, tamed versions of HIV, small-pox, and measles) to kill cancer cells: *Killing Cancer*.[1] It's experimental now, and the treatment currently seems far more aggressive and dangerous than standard chemotherapy, but the trick of taking a deadly virus and redesigning it to kill only cancer cells, by entering and replicating until the cancer cell literally explodes, is awe-inspiringly clever. At Mayo and MD Anderson, for example, multiple myeloma and childhood leukemia have both been successfully cured by the virus treatment. The documentary made me weep, not only for the patients, whose fear, pain, and ultimate triumph over cancer is so touching, but also for the researchers whose funds for cancer research dried up after the 2008 financial collapse, itself caused by the old metaphorical cancer of greed that, just like the real thing, seems inevitable.

I'm not scouring the Internet for information on cancer anymore, but even so I occasionally stumble on some new promising research, such as that which has recently found that it is possible to starve cancer cells, and cancer cells only, of nutrients. This research is very much still in the lab, but it sounds like great news because the potential therapy would have none of the side effects of conventional cancer treatment—surgical, chemotherapeutic, or otherwise. Specifically, the new molecule developed for treatment prevents autophagy, which is sort of the last-ditch effort of cancer to survive—eating itself when all other energy sources have been denied.[2]

Regardless of the unpredictability of tomorrow's cancer treatments, it's impossible for me not to think about the future occasionally, by which I mean maybe ten to twenty times during any given day. I can normally bring myself back to my blind spot in time, the real present, with a stubborn, mulish insistence on focusing on the present moment, even though it can't be seen. My psychotherapist explained, quite convincingly, that the best strategy for handling my future cancer treatment is to forget about it and leave it to my oncologist. Because that's *his* job.

So I'm gradually, almost imperceptibly, moving my blind spots, my scotomata, to the future.

My psychotherapist, who is in his seventies, skis, sometimes at the same mountain resort that I go to. Last week at the end of our session, I asked him which were his favorite runs there. He said he didn't really have any favorites because they were all "too groomed, too tamed." He likes the chutes, he says. These chutes are only for advanced skiers, if you know what's good for you. They are decidedly ungroomed, rough, boulder strewn and, to my mind, dangerous. Every few years someone is killed in the chutes on a mountain somewhere in the United States. I vaguely remember that the last person I heard about being killed was a young expert skier who misjudged a jump. The back of his head bounced back and off a boulder, killing him instantly.

I stared at my psychotherapist in slack-jawed wonder. He said he likes the chutes because if you ski them, you can't think about anything but the present moment. "The second you think about something other than what you are doing that very moment, the mountain will take you." As shocking as this revelation was to me, it is familiar. Heather has her mindfulness. I have my motorcycle.

Heather Responds to
"My Blind Spots"

This is the kind of thing that he does—take a perfectly reasonable and useful therapeutic or meditation practice and turn it into a linguistic problem, as if recasting the problem into the well-worn grooves of language will solve it—here specifically fear of the future and inability to focus on the present. I don't fault him for the worry. I'm worried. But I meditate to deal with it. Meditation is too woo-woo for him. (Either that or too boring.) Is it that Texas ethos that makes it hard to take the rational route to enlightenment? Don is always looking for answers in all the hard places. Or is it a guy thing? But at least half of the people in my meditation group are men. His psychotherapist is far from a Texan. And he recommends meditation to his patients. I know because I've seen him several times myself. Yet he goes to the chutes to escape his mind? I don't even know why I wonder about this. So I guess it's just a strategy that some people use—danger (climbing radio towers, jumping off railroad trestles, skiing chutes) is a time-honored way of being with the self without the "chattering monkey" of interior voices.

Mental extremes can work as well, I think. Don rarely turns to physical danger to silence these other voices. He does ride his homemade motorcycle, which to me would be akin to building your own rocket ship. One blown O-ring on takeoff on the highway and you're toast. And he does sometimes do stuff like climb fourteeners in Colorado or go on long bike rides without training for them, after he's been sitting on his ass writing for six months. But most of the time he'll use a brain challenge to concentrate on—computer programming, teaching himself X, Y, or Z when it would be so much easier to just take a meditation class or philosophize and turn mortality into a contrived problem of tense in language analysis.

I am glad that Don finally saw his psychotherapist. I had been urging him to do so since last summer. It's typical of Don to take my suggestions belatedly so that to him they seem like his own idea. I felt compelled to remind him that I had been urging him to see the therapist all these months because he came back so proud of himself and relieved after his session. I remind him of this, not to lord it over him, but rather in the hope that he will take my often sound advice sooner rather than later the next time he needs a good kick in the psychological pants. But I'm pretty sure this is a vain hope because unless he's in physical pain, Don is more likely to sit around like some German metaphysician trying to *think* his way through the analysis and synthesis of his problem. It's a hard way to live, but that's who he is.

Notes

1. VICE *Special Report: Killing Cancer.* YouTube and HBO now charge for the documentary. When I first watched it in 2015, it was free of charge.

2. Fikes, "New Approaches to Starving Cancers."

Letting Go

March 28

M Y LAST WEEK OF CHEMO, two weeks ago, began like all the rest except for the rather obvious smirk on my face that said, "I'm almost done with this and I ain't never gonna study chemo no more." I was convinced that I knew exactly what I was in for, familiar as I was with the process after having gone through it five times already: three days of steadily decreasing energy and increasing fog from the chemo, followed by the dreaded pegfilgrastim injection and then feeling sick as a dog for at least four days and then feeling sick as a cat for the rest of the week. It was spring break at the university, and on the first day, I asked the infusion nurse who mixes and fills the infusion bags to put a tiny paper umbrella on mine. I should have thought ahead and brought my own. She was willing but, alas, fresh out of cocktail umbrellas. In the middle of it all, a friend said it must help knowing this was the last chemo treatment, and it did help, both knowing that and hearing it from my dear friend, who has been a solid pen pal through this whole experience. She apologized unnecessarily for not e-mailing me sometime in the middle of the treatment week, saying that she had intended to on Tuesday but Fred, their dog (my second favorite dog in the whole world even though we know each other only through Facebook and e-mail), ate an entire bag of shit that evening. It probably didn't affect him the way it would me, but the chemo flu, which is as slow to come out of as the real flu, feels like I ate a big bag of shit with all kinds of unhealthy bacteria in it. These are the kinds of thoughts I have in the midst of chemo flu: "I wonder where Fred found this bag of shit, just in case I want to appreciate the gift of life, say, six months from now, and I'm all like, 'Fuck this job, fuck my mortgage, fuck my life, I'm gonna eat a bag of shit and die.'" It wouldn't kill me, but it would remind me of everything I have to be thankful for.

And then, just like that, chemo is over. Anyone who has been through six months of chemotherapy at my cancer center knows that on the last day of chemotherapy, no matter how long you've been in treatment, you get to ring the bell. They have two: a cowbell, which doesn't seem appropriate to me, and a church hand bell, much more to my liking. The sound is high and clear. I'd heard it many times before. You can't help but cheer when someone rings it. My cheering became more and more enthusiastic the closer I got to the end of treatment myself. On Monday of my last week, the bell rang and I snapped out of a comfortable Benadryl cloud to cheer as if I were at a Fourth of July parade of local war veterans, a few with missing limbs, a few in wheelchairs, but all so shockingly heroic and noble you just have to weep. It was exhilarating to whoop and clap and yell and cry a little too.

There are all manner of inappropriate and unkind thoughts one can have in chemo, or at least I did. Chemo lasted seven and a half hours on Monday of my last week. It was like a real job. Two infusion nurses were out sick, and bless their hearts for staying home. And the two that were on duty were overwhelmed with everyone's neediness and drip lines all going dry at the same time and so on. I didn't mind the extra time at all, really; it was only about an hour longer than usual. The woman in chemo in the cubicle next to mine was talking loudly, nonstop, about nothing anybody other than she would be interested in, as if yelling it all out would make it more interesting to everyone. I'm pretty sure I'm right about this because that's how I lecture in classes. I stubbornly figure that the louder I get, the more interesting what I have to say will seem to the class. I can go from silence to make-'em-jump-out-of-their-seats in an instant. I do normally apologize and calm it down a bit when I make someone flinch. And really, I'm never yelling anything as important or content-filled as "Fire!" A typical high-decibel pronouncement might be "This distillation of all syntactic rules to essentially three very abstract algebraic-like rules is one of the most awesome things about the human mind that I know of."[1] I not only yell, I repeat, ad nauseam, as if volume and repetition, so essential to rock music, will make me sound profound or cool or something. I can't remember where the woman's rambling story was going, but some of the details included "I need to call nephew so-and-so, I haven't heard from him and his new wife since that wedding, I think my bowels are in an uproar, is there any of that cake left from last night, I didn't like those cupcakes at all, I thought that icing was just weird, though I wouldn't tell Betty that for anything, but I really couldn't get through more than one, I just left that part of that second one on my plate and nobody said anything, poor thing was nice to try in the first place, don't you think? . . ." About four hours into the day, the woman lost her voice and thought she was *dying*. The nurses put her on oxygen, I don't know, because maybe it couldn't hurt and maybe because it would keep her quiet. My theory is that she had just worn her voice out.

Everybody knows chemo weakens both your thoracic diaphragm, making breathing more and more shallow, and your abdominal muscles, which then in turn cannot expel the decreasing volume of air with sufficient force to produce normal speech. All of this is why no one can do anything but whisper from about the third morning on. Or at least that's the way it is with me, every single time. This is why you should try to conserve your strength. The vocal folds themselves are tensed for speech by muscles that can be weakened by chemo. When the woman lost her voice, I was tempted to pop my head up over the dividing glass between our cubicles and give her a two-hour informative steroid-fueled completely free lecture on the physiology of speech. She had a friend with her who didn't have cancer and therefore could fill up the remainder of the seven and a half hours with chatter. Her friend sounded kind of relieved to finally get her turn in the conversation, beyond the occasional "uh-huh" and "you don't say" that her friend with cancer had allowed her. She mostly complained about what sounded like an entirely different set of thankless relatives. This second set really did seem awful.

By Wednesday, when the time came for me to ring the church hand bell six times, once for each of my months of treatment, I felt like Slim Pickens swinging his cowboy hat and riding the bomb into oblivion in *Dr. Strangelove.*

I reproduce some memorable quotations from my nurses, not all of which I heard. Heather was there and reported some:

"You're a rock star, Don."

"You made it look easy!"

"And I thought I was going to scare you away"—this from the intake orientation nurse, with whom I've traded endless documentary recommendations. She's a big Jack White fan, which I am too. Her favorite Pandora station is blues and blues rock, which they were playing on Wednesday. So on that last day, until it got crowded, it was bliss to hear Jimi Hendrix, Led Zeppelin, White Stripes, Lightnin' Hopkins, Junior Kimbrough . . . It felt like home. Just when I was about to leave. Hopefully for good.

All my nurses are so incredibly kind. Their job would put a callus on me an inch thick in one week. Lord, I'm going to miss them.

On Thursday I got the usual pegfilgrastim injection. Took about five minutes, including the waiting room time. The nurse who gave it to me knew it was my last week. She gave me a hug for good luck and good health.

Friday, the chemo flu put me in bed for about twenty hours, the four missing hours spent peeing. Saturday was worse, Sunday was worse still, Monday was as yet the cruelest day, including something new, a headache that no safe amount of Advil, Aleve, or

Tylenol would banish, even into the vaguest directions of a corner. I slept with frozen ice packs on the crown of my skull, alternating with ice packs on my forehead, although never both at once because I kept imagining my brain freezing to the consistency of a slushie. I had an ice chest filled with about six such packs—my ice packs had ice packs to keep them frozen until I melted them, and I was running a fever of 101.9 degrees all night as well. My digital thermometer is kindly provided by the company that makes the pegfilgrastim that I take. The company name is all over the very nice thermometer case. I kept imagining a conversation something like the following taking place in, say, a moderately loud bowling alley.

"Hey, that's a nifty thermometer!"

"Thanks, really, thanks."

"You don't look so good, dude. Are you sure you should be lying in the middle of a bowling alley with an ice pack on your head taking your temperature?"

"No, man, I'm great! The company that gave me this thermometer makes the white blood cell growth protein that gives me the fever and headache that is making me want to rip my face off just now. I'm here because I'm checking out what hell might feel and sound like."

My temperature had fallen to 99 point something by six in the morning, which is a time when I never, ever get up unless I have a blinding headache or some other chemo-induced madness. I managed to choke down some oatmeal and the ever-important water. My appointment with my oncologist was for 10:00 a.m. Heather and I were on time.

The blood test was fine, with no mention that I was dehydrated, the case according to the metabolic panel I had taken on Monday. I did tell my onc about extreme fatigue and the headaches. He said something entirely logical about alternating Tylenol and Advil in very careful ways, according to Heather. What I heard was, "Ahhh, you can take Tylenol in addition to Advil if you take Advil for twenty-four hours and if in the last dose only you take Tylenol but before you take Advil again and you don't look so good, Don. Stick out your tongue." I did that. He pronounced me dehydrated and told me to drink water, which I was holding a bottle of at that moment, so I was happy to oblige.

Heather had several questions we had planned to ask but which I wasn't up to understanding just then, like, which medications should he take for how much longer and when do you want to see him again and blah, blah, blah? How long do the chemotherapy drugs stay in his system? No, seriously? During these important questions, I had lain back down on the examining table because I had neither the strength nor the dignity to sit up on the edge of the table. My oncologist left, saying good-bye and that I didn't look so good but all the blood tests did and to take care. Two important timing details have to be pointed out here. First, I had never seen him for follow-up as early as a Tuesday. A day can make a dramatic difference in how one feels after chemo. Second, the side effects of the chemo and pegfilgrastim were clearly worse than they had ever been before, which is entirely to be expected. It will now take at least six months to clear all the toxic drugs that have been pumped into my body through the port in my chest for the past six months. Kind of like getting over a messy breakup.

After my oncologist left, I raised myself to a sitting position, pushing back a wave of nausea. I told Heather that I was feeling nauseated. She left the room to see whether she could locate a nurse or my oncologist to give me an anti-emetic. I fell to my knees and rested my head on the seat of the chair Heather had been sitting in and then pulled myself up to a semi-sitting posture because it just seemed undignified to be found kneeling from nausea and weakness. Heather came back in and said something that I cannot remember at all about anti-emetics. I was slumped over with elbows on knees, spilling the water left in the bottle.

Heather said, "Don, you're spilling water everywhere!"

"Okay," I agreed, and then I tried wiping some of it up with a gauze pad my nurse had given me when he took the blood sample.

"Don't worry about that, Don." That's the last I remember before . . .

"*Don! Don! Wake up! Wake up! Don! Are you there?!*" The words were muffled, as if my head were wrapped in a warm wet blanket. And someone was shaking me and pulling on me. Heather told me later that I had sat up after trying to clean up the water, my head had fallen back against the window, my face had gone white as milk, and my eyes had both rolled back in my head so that nothing showed but the whites.

I remember almost nothing of the experience except being half awake and that five of the nurses I knew were in the room, all yelling at me to wake up. I woke up just enough to say, "I don't know what happened."

"We need to get him back on the table."

"How are we going to get him back on the table?"

"There are enough of us that we can probably lift him."

"*Don, wake up!* Stay with us. Help us move you to the bed. Can you do that?"

"Yeah." And two of them got under each shoulder, another pushed from behind, and a fourth pulled.

Once on the table, I slurred, "I'm okay, but I don't know what happened."

"You fainted, Don. You *have* to stay awake!"

I fell asleep—or passed out, it seems—at least three more times. Each time, I was startled back to semi-consciousness with "Don, stay awake! Stay with us! *Do you hear me, Don?*"

Somebody slipped an oxygen tube around my neck and up my nostrils, which helped a bit, but I still kept passing out. Then I felt somebody rip up my shirt and start rubbing really hard on my sternum. "Yep, here it is," I thought, "the heart attack." Instead, this person, whom I couldn't really see because my eyes were still rolling around, was digging into my sternum with a fist that felt like it was sheathed in a welding glove. I had rarely felt such pain before. I woke up fast and pretty much stayed awake because the next thing one of my favorite nurses did (now I could see who was there and closest) was lean far over me with an access needle for my port and insert it with no anesthetic. I had time to think, "Access port. Needle. No anesthetic." Now I was completely awake and screaming with the pain from my sternum rub and the jab in my access port. I can remember watching my right leg do a high kick in horizontal position. The wet blanket feeling was gone.

By the time the pulsing pain from my sternum and port started to abate, I was beginning to feel close to normal. I kind of took a wobbly look around the room. I knew all the nurses there very well, by my current rough estimate then about six. Heather and one of the nurses were at the far end of the room hugging, and Heather was sobbing. That scared me and then I started to cry.

The nurse closest to the bed said, "What's wrong?"

"Nothing, just a little emotional."

"That's okay. You're okay. You're awake again."

Then, with no transition whatsoever, as if I was the least skilled conversationalist in the world, I turned to my nurse friend who shares my enthusiasm for Jack White and said loudly, "Have you seen the concert with Jack White and Robert Plant doing Zeppelin songs on YouTube?"

I didn't hear or process the response, but Heather said later that she and the nurses started laughing and someone said, "Well, he's definitely back!"

"Jack White has almost as good a blues voice as Robert Plant!" I went on.

My buddy said she'd check it out.

In the meantime someone had rustled up the EMTs (it's protocol), who strongly suggested but did not insist that I be taken to a hospital to be checked out. Heather and I agreed that this was a good call. Before we left, one took vitals, while the other made notes and asked questions. The latter noticed the water on the floor and the front of my pants, and absently murmured, "Incontinent." I didn't protest. The EMT who sat in the back of the ambulance with me and I swapped jokes all the way across town. Her best: "I'm going to get you an ocean-front view." I laughed. She said that she was impressed that I got it. I suspect it was yet another clever test.

Seven hours later, fully rested and hydrated, and cleared with a CT scan of my heart and lungs for blood clots, I was released into the wild. The best way I've found to get medical information is to ask nurses. My ER nurse, the nicest guy you'd ever want to meet, said that what was performed on me to wake me is called a "sternal rub." He said it's one of approximately three ways medical professionals have of determining whether someone is "still with us or not."

What I found extraordinary about the experience was how easy it was letting go and how hard it was coming back. I don't think my life was ever in serious danger (considering that I was cleared of the primary danger of blood clots; my oncologist pronounced that I had simply vagaled down), but if the moment of death is simply the turning off of the light, even if the light flickers, in a sudden or step-wise letting go of the world, this little mini-experience was easeful. The return to the world of consciousness and love and relative good health was and is as sweet and loud and insistent as the thousands of pink and white crabapple and pear trees in blossom that pull at the eye and perfume the air this time of year, even if for just a short while.

Heather Responds to "Letting Go"

Never mind that this easeful passage to unconsciousness is not a typical way to pass into death. There was nothing about this experience that was easeful to me, I'll tell you that.

It is true that Don will probably miss his nurses. But he'll get over that. We've talked before about how all his nurses see hundreds of patients in a year, and they have different experiences and relationships with all of them. Most friendships are not meant to last for a lifetime. I have friends who date back to college, but I talk to them just a couple of times a year. One of my friends went through breast cancer surgery and chemotherapy and didn't tell me until afterward. Her way of dealing with cancer was to try to ignore it as best as she could. Don's way has been to make a hobby of it: reading and writing about cancer and the latest treatments, writing this book, and trying his best to stay informed about his particular treatments. And, perhaps as important as anything else, maintaining friendly relationships with his nurses and doctors. It's hard not to respect nurses and doctors, but Don grew to like them as people as well. He thinks it is almost inconceivable that someone would choose to practice oncology except in the context of laboratory research. This is one reason why he finds his nurses and doctors fascinating—they practice a branch of medicine that is one of the most challenging and interesting intellectually but must be one of the most heartbreaking personally.

How do you handle a career in a medical specialty that by its nature features a relatively high incidence of mortality? Back when both Don and I lived in Texas and both suffered from seasonal allergies seriously enough to take allergen injections once a week, one of our fellow allergy sufferers said that allergists have the best of all possible physician specialties: their patients rarely die, but then again they never get well either.

In any case, this scare that put Don in the emergency room for a day reminds me yet again of how much is at stake in his cancer treatment. We've been married for over thirty years. I haven't put up with this guy for all this time just to have him abandon me for death now. We both have decided to retire next academic year. I will in December. Don will a semester later in June. These decisions took quite a bit of careful planning, although all that figuring, calculation of numbers (some of which Don did himself in determining what our expenses were for last year), and reassurance from our financial counselors don't prevent Don from dwelling on his lifelong fear that he will end up living in a truck. He talks about it so much I sometimes think that's what he would actually prefer. But we did do all the planning and calculating. Barring unforeseeable global economic ruin, we are good for retirement, even and especially if Don survives his cancer and dies from something much more prosaic, like crashing his dumbass motorcycle. He says he wants to write full-time. I don't really care what he does—write, ride his motorcycle or bicycle, fish, or play one of his many guitars—as long as he doesn't die doing it. It would be nice to keep the emergency room visits to a minimum too. Don will turn sixty this July. In preparation he's been practicing yelling, "Hey, punks, get off my lawn!" Don's always looking for ways to make new friends.

Notes

1. An extraordinarily clear introduction to this theory of language structure can be found in Andrew Carnie's *Syntax*.

Fuck Cancer!

April 8

I'M THREE WEEKS OUT from my last chemo treatment. My onc pulled me off acyclovir (an anti-viral) a week ago because he suspected it was causing my fevers of over 101 degrees. He was right. Now I'm back on acyclovir, for one day so far now, because my immune system will be seriously compromised for about six months, and I still need it along with an anti-bacterial. So far, so good: no fever yet. I'm keeping the port for at least three months "just in case" I turn out to be one of the unlucky ones whose remission fails quickly. But it's just in case, and I am not looking forward to having it removed when the time comes. Surely I can talk my surgeon into prescribing something a bit stronger than Tylenol for the procedure. Until I have it removed, I must have it cleared once a month. I still have half a tube of lidocaine, with which I intend to obsessively slather the skin covering my port every single time since I now know what it feels like to have that port accessed without anesthetic. I'm still not sleeping well, but I haven't slept well for so long that it seems like the new normal. I unfailingly wake up after five to six hours of sleep, when I used to need eight or nine hours of uninterrupted sleep to feel human. On most days I take an hour nap in the afternoon, especially if I've been Skyped in for a committee meeting or two in my department. I suspect my sleep is getting imperceptibly better, but I still experience surreal, inexplicable, and hard-to-remember nightmares almost every night.

I never dream anymore that I show up in my underwear to teach my classes. Instead, one frequent nightmare I can remember—because it's one I had occasionally as a child—is being chased through an apocalyptic landscape by a sharply spiked metal ball the size of a two-story house. I don't know what that spiky metal ball meant to me as a child, although I was terrified of it, and that terror usually lasted well into the day after I had that particular nightmare. Now it seems rather obvious to me that it's a nasty-ass cancer cell trying to catch and impale me. I suspect that the fear of cancer will fade some over time, even if the statistical threat doesn't. At one time my greatest fear was chemotherapy; now I'm not afraid of it at all. Which doesn't mean I like it; it just doesn't scare me. So the next time I startle myself awake embarrassed that I walked into a syntax class in nothing but my boxers and wool socks, I'll know that I'm completely normal again.

I'm seeing my favorite dermatologist later today. After she examines all my moles and warts and general imperfections with her jeweler's loupe, I'm going to ask her if there is any emergency (cosmetic) surgery that I need or even that she can imagine that I'll ever need, because I've met my insurance deductible this year and even maxed out on out-of-pocket medical costs. I look at recent photos friends have taken of me, and it seems to me that I look older than my fifty-nine, almost sixty, years. My theory is that the chemotherapy has aged me prematurely and that that's just not right or fair in America. Maybe if I get gobs of Botox injections I can develop a poker face and start supplementing my income at the local casinos. It probably will come in handy for faculty and committee meetings as well when I start having to show up in person. Now when I Skype in, I just upload my latest attempt at humor, for example, a photo of Bubbles from *Trailer Park Boys* dressed as "The Green Bastard." Just as I floss and brush my teeth obsessively before a dental appointment, I thoroughly lubricate myself with SPF15 body moisturizing lotion this morning. If my dermatologist even suggests anything cutty or gougy today, I'm going to be harder to hold onto than a greased miniature potbellied pig.

Oh, and I probably don't have prostate cancer, a fear that I've been living with for a couple of months since my first checkup with my new urologist, who discovered a high PSA count. I saw my urologist again last week. He pronounced my latest PSA levels normal. Said I might want to have one (or two, if I'm worried) PSA tests per year. I kept a straight face except for expressing profound thanks until I got outside. Then I leaped and danced and yodeled in the parking lot, howling at Mount Rose, sitting right there in front of me to the west looking exactly like itself, only bigger and more magnificent. The threat of the possible need for a prostate biopsy and then the possibility of needing more chemo or even radiation for prostate cancer had been weighing me down for a couple of weeks since I had started to recover from the last CLL/SLL chemotherapy treatment. It felt like the threat of having to serve two back-to-back life sentences. I get to the end of one seemingly interminable treatment cycle, and the judge says, "Oh, you very bad boy, back to chemo with you. This time I hope you learn your lesson."

As I wrote earlier, PSA (prostate-specific antigen) is not a terribly accurate test for prostate cancer, but it's practically the only test urologists have other than a biopsy. I've read that only 25 percent of men with elevated PSA turn out to have prostate cancer on biopsy, which you don't want to hear about, although of course I would have written a chapter with all the hell of it in high definition if I'd had high PSA in the latest test.[1] PSA can be elevated for all kinds of reasons, most of which involve a prostate that is agitato because of any number of possible causes: prostate digital exams themselves; riding a bicycle; having a urinary tract infection; having prostatitis; and, of course, prostate cancer itself.[2] I've read studies claiming that pomegranate juice lowers PSA levels.[3] I'm drinking pomegranate juice like strawberry wine now, although I know that's magical thinking because high PSA levels are not the disease, they are simply sometimes a symptom of the disease. It seems to my nonmedical mind to be similar to obsessively eating cough drops to treat a smoker's cough. Mostly I just like the taste of pomegranate juice. Somebody named Oprah, maybe even *the* Oprah, apparently has a favorite pomegranate martini recipe.[4]

My normal life is slowing coming back to me in both clarity and strength. The better I feel each day, the more newly grateful I am that my doctors and nurses have somehow managed to save my life so far. For the time being, I try not to think about how much time and money it all took or that the cancer is guaranteed to return someday. I hope only that it's sometime in the very distant future. I'm very grateful to my university for the partial leave it gave me (from all teaching duties) so that I could stay safe. I would have been useless in the classroom anyway, except for entertaining students with rambling, disconnected stories about chemotherapy and then slumping at my desk.

This is how normal my life is now. I spent most of this past Saturday trying to change out the starter ring gear on my motorcycle. The starter ring gear was shrieking like a chainsaw attempting to cut through a metal fence post about every fifth time I tried to start the bike. This noise gives people good reason to hate bikers and me in particular. This noise is awful. The problem is that somehow a few of the teeth on the starter ring gear got themselves shredded, probably because of a poorly adjusted starter pinion gear. Turns out that getting the old starter gear off the clutch basket wasn't that big a problem. All it took was several hours of Internet research, an acetylene torch to heat the ring, half a can of WD40, a good large rubber mallet, and some well-placed whacks to wooden slats placed to absorb some of but transmit most of the force to the ring. The ring is sitting here on the floor of my study reminding me of how much fun I had taking it off the clutch basket. The problem now will be getting a new one on. I'll have to freeze the clutch basket in our freezer, without telling Heather, for several hours while simultaneously heating the new starter ring gear in our oven for several hours, again without telling Heather, and then I'll have to introduce them to one another in their opposing thermal states and hope that they mate successfully for life.

I'm grateful to friends, relatives, colleagues, and students who shopped for us, cooked delicious meals for us, accompanied me to appointments when Heather couldn't, sent gifts and cards of support, e-mailed encouraging notes, telephoned to check up on us, showed love and inspired gratitude in me every day, and looked after Heather when I couldn't. I'm also very grateful to colleagues who picked up my service commitments when I just couldn't meet a deadline during a down week and who Skyped me into committee and faculty meetings that I couldn't attend in person.

I'm most grateful to Heather, who checked and double-checked all the details of my treatment, did practically all out-of-house duties to keep the house running, sat with me when I was too sick to hold my head up, including spending all day with me at the hospital just two weeks ago, and somehow managed to keep doing her impossibly hard job at the university through it all. And she also somehow contained her fear all these months so as not to increase my own.

Years ago one of our best lawyers told us that the soundest financial advice she could give us was not to get divorced. Not that we've even come close to divorcing or even thinking about it. It just seems inconceivable. As both Heather and I get nearer retirement age and start looking at our financial condition for retirement, I'm pretty sure I understand the money side of the advice. I also think I now realize the wisdom of that part of traditional wedding vows in which each swears to love the other in sickness and in health. I don't think it's easier to love someone in a marriage when one of the partners is sick, but I do know that the love changes and matures during that time in ways that I couldn't have predicted. Gratitude, both on the part of the partner who receives care and support and on the part of the one who is threatened but spared devastating loss, is a powerful bond. About devastating loss, that storm toward which we are all sailing and through which some of my friends and relatives have already sailed, I know nothing. The only state I can possibly imagine in my ignorance is stunned silence and bottomless grief, perhaps ultimately tempered by a deeper appreciation of the mysteries of both life and death.

I've heard that publishers suffer something like chemo nausea when they see a cancer survivor headed their way lugging a manuscript. I'll try to be sympathetic. I think I have two or three unused professional barf bags left over from hospital stays.

Two days ago I ordered the biggest box of the best-quality brownies I know about on the Internet or anywhere else (Fairytale Brownies) as a thank-you for my oncology practice, especially for looking after me and Heather during my fainting spell the last time I was in.[5] The box will be delivered tomorrow. These brownies have no narcotics in them except some really, really fine chocolate. Nevertheless, the quality of these truly amazing brownies is such that the next time I visit my onc, I expect to find everyone lying around in pajamas and bathrobes, munching on brownies with heavy-lidded eyes.

One of my students sent me a gift through Heather's office. It wasn't wrapped, so Heather peeked to see what it was. Her personnel specialist rides a Harley-Davidson and knew exactly what it was—a Harley demon bell, a small silver bell usually attached to the underside of one's motorcycle to keep the road demons away. This one had some small engraving on it: on one side "Don Hardy, 1; CLL/SLL, 0," and on the other "Fuck Cancer!"

Heather Responds to
"Fuck Cancer!"

I don't think I'd seen Don happier in the last year than when his urologist said his PSA was normal. I had been telling him since the high results came in from the first test to try not to worry about it, that the test was unreliable, etc. But he was worried, and it was an immense relief to get the all clear from the urologist.

Don is extraordinarily proud of his "Fuck Cancer" Harley bell. He's changed his unofficial name on Facebook to Harley Bell, complete with an automatically generated sound file for help in pronunciation. He thinks this is funny. Sigh.

He is most proud, I think, that a student of his went to the trouble and thought to give him this gift. I am thankful too.

What I find fascinating is the "Fuck Cancer" meme. I think I know how it is supposed to be taken, as an insult to Cancer, as if Cancer, personified and capitalized, is a human being that you can speak ill of in the third person. There are all sorts of interesting variations one could imagine for this insult. "Fuck you, Cancer": here the victim or friend or loved one speaks directly to Cancer. That is a bit bold, though. Do you want to insult Cancer to its face? Or there's "Fuck. Cancer," which sounds like a declaration of dismay, as in "Fuck me. Candidate X won the election." "Fuck, Cancer" sounds like the internal voice of a cancer victim on first hearing the diagnosis. "Fuck Cancer" is just ambiguous enough to be useful for expressing a variety of common thoughts I've had about cancer in the last year. There is the aggressive "Fuck Cancer," as in "I hate cancer and am inclined to believe that there are so few friends of cancer out there that I'm likely to get away with an otherwise questionably socially acceptable epithet." I recently saw a "Fuck Cancer" T-shirt on a guy in a store; he told me that he bought it from a biker club selling them to raise money for victims. There is also the "Fuck Cancer" as in "Fuck work. I'm going fishing." This is probably the best interpretation since cancer cannot be insulted, and we can shape only our own feelings. There was little room or time for this "Fuck Cancer" attitude this year, given how sick the chemotherapy made Don. But now he and I have an opportunity to "Fuck Cancer" and "Go Fishing." He hasn't gone fishing yet, probably only because we are in the middle of a seven-year drought here in Nevada. But he is bicycling and playing his guitars again, both of which I take to be good signs. He's also taken to reading detective fiction, which he would never read before because he was too busy reading "serious fiction" for his work. This I take to be another way of saying "Fuck Cancer."

As for the gift of brownies to the staff at his oncologist's practice, this is only the latest example of Don going too far in thanking people. I can't tell you the number of extravagant gifts I've talked Don out of giving this year to friends, colleagues, and the oncology staff. It seems to be his way not only of expressing gratitude but of taking a more active role, since the chemotherapy laid him so low for so long. This is probably a good time for me to get neglected repair jobs done around the house. Practically the first things he did when he could stay out of bed for eight hours at a time were replace the broken lock and fix the air-conditioning on his Jeep, both of which have been broken for the last five years. I was impressed.

Notes

1. "Prostate-Specific Antigen (psa) Test."
2. Iliades, "What a High psa Level Means if It's Not Prostate Cancer"; "What Is Prostatitis?"
3. Castle, "Pomegranate Juice."
4. "Oprah's Favorite Pomegranate Martini Recipe."
5. "Brownies by Fairytale."

Watching but Not Waiting

April 20

I SEE MY ONCOLOGIST tomorrow for my first official post-chemo-therapy blood analysis. He will be watching for signs of a probably slow but inexorable rise in my white blood cell count or growth in the remaining lymph nodes in my armpits or in my neck or anywhere else. Honestly, I don't know how quickly oncologists act when "remission starts to fail," still an odd and oxymoronic phrase to my mind. It will probably come up in conversation tomorrow.

In another sense I'm not waiting. Both Heather and I are talking with our financial planner this week about retirement. Heather has simply worked herself to the point of exhaustion being dean here at UNR, facing budget cuts that would make four-star generals in the Department of Defense weep like three-year-olds and dealing with personnel problems that make Obama's relationship with the Republicans and the Tea Partyers look like a sixties love-in. The longer you are dean the harder life gets, especially at a time when Nevada's state legislature, like most these days, looks to slash funding for higher education to make its pathetically underfunded budget limp its way into the next legislative session. It is the dean who must make hard decisions when money is scarce. And hard decisions always piss somebody off, especially in a university.

I'm hoping to retire next summer, which will put my time in higher education at thirty-five years, although a number of those years were spent in servitude as a graduate teaching assistant. Those early years were the hardest; it's good that I was young when I went through them. And before 1980 I spent seven years off and on in full-time, part-time, and summer jobs, first living the third-shift blue-collar dream and then living the just as sleep-deprived life of an undergraduate student.

Before the cancer, I told friends—and I believed it—that I would work at least until I was seventy-five. But then I was counting on at least eighty-five pretty good years in this life. Now that I have a disease in which the treatment I just went through has an average remission span of six and a half years,[1] I'm convinced that thirty-five years in the job is more than enough, especially since the chemotherapy, like the shoulder surgeries and the subsequent physical therapy, has essentially derailed my research and writing projects. Research and writing require prolonged concentration, something that is damned near impossible if you are spending two weeks out of every month sick in bed and sleeping more than twelve hours a day just to escape the pain for a while.

So I'm going to fish, I'm going to write, I'm going to sit down by the river with Lyle. Heather and I are going to explore all of the western United States before it all dries up and just blows away in the wind someday.

I can hardly believe that if I get my wish and both Heather and I are able to retire sometime in the next year, I will most likely have a little more than a year left to work. That seems like a long time since so much can happen in the life of a cancer patient in a year. The secret to getting through this year happily is, I think, to apply all the lessons that I've imperfectly learned with so much pain and discomfort and worry over the past ten months: live in the present, enjoy the present if at all possible, and if it's not possible, then change your life, habits, or ways of thinking so that you *can* enjoy the present, because the present is the only thing you have. And the truth that makes the present too precious for language, really, is that any present moment—that experience of being in the present, being in time—can be ripped away, sometimes with no warning whatsoever. Or I may get a few months' warning. But however much or little warning I get, it will be someday, probably sooner rather than the much later that I've always hoped for, that the life, the consciousness, the memory, the pleasures, the ones I love, will all either be taken away from me or I from them.

If I haven't always lived the examined life, I certainly am now. I've taught all I can teach. I've served on all the committees I can serve on. Now, it is time to reap whatever fruit or grains have resulted from thirty-five years of working and studying in the university, another five years as an undergraduate student, and twenty years as a child, a bumbling adolescent, and a clueless young adult. I've always wanted to be a full-time writer.

I've happily spent my career concerned more about my students and teaching than anything. That enthusiasm, luck, excellent students, and working in great departments explain the three university-wide teaching awards I've won. I'm moving into the retirement period of my life, but retirement doesn't just mean fishing. It means having time for those things that you love—like writing—that you've never taken proper time for. This is going to be a hoot.

Heather Responds to
"Watching but Not Waiting"

I've always told him that he can write. I knew that when he wrote me from graduate school in Houston while I was working in Denton. His letters are funny and tender, and I still treasure them. As Don pulls out of the spiral of pain and disorientation and despair of the last year, I can see his energy returning, but it is redirected. I can tell that he really doesn't want to go back for another year of teaching, although he feels he owes it to the department not to retire without at least a semester's notice. Friends of his have been very kind to him this year and taken up many of the duties, including overload teaching, to make up for his absence.

Don has already done what he can to prepare for the transition to retired life and work. Aside from this book on his own cancer, he has one more academic book planned, but he'd like that one to be a crossover book about the self in the popular American imagination. And he has other writing plans, including becoming an indie self-published mystery writer. He's been reading up on the genre this summer and even working through a police procedural book. He has a very slight chance of making pocket change as a self-published writer, but I have warned him about possible failure. Failure doesn't seem to be a concern. He's more interested in learning something new and bringing a new challenge to his life that might draw on an existing gift, the ability to write.

Not everybody can write. And not everyone who can write can write fiction. Don has spent his academic life writing both abstract and empirically based articles and books on syntax, semantics, pragmatics, and stylistics (that last being the linguistic analysis of literature). It's a rarefied topic for a small, specialized audience. And even though many people have at one time been told or thought to themselves that they have a book in them, few people have books that they can get out of them, especially fiction. But Don likes a challenge.

Notes
1. "Is Long-Term Remission with FCR a Cure?"

On Not Being the
Center of the Universe

May 26

ITHINK EVERYTHING is about as back to normal as it will ever be.
I haven't even had my first three-month remission check, but
the nodes aren't swelling. I have residual fatigue and the return of
what I called the cancer acne, but I'm beginning to suspect that it,
like my Peyronie's bent dick, is not a result of the cancer at all but
part of the effects of aging, or allergies, or God knows what.

Yesterday, I went on an epic big grocery run at one of those
huge stores that politically correct people don't shop at and I came
back wheezing and breathing hard. But this morning I'm going
on my first long bicycle ride since the cancer treatment, a ride on
level terrain down by the river, away from the hills that stretch in
all directions from my house so that it is impossible to go on even
a short ride from there without wishing I had a personal stash of
steroids.

In a lot of ways, my life has been more interesting over the last
year than over the many previous decades. I think there is a reason
for the widespread rumor that active combat makes people feel
more alive than they ever have before. That which is about to be
taken from you, life, becomes more precious, it seems. I've never
been in battle, but I have made more resolutions in the last year
than in my whole life: to be kinder, to enjoy each day, to finish this
or that book, to learn music theory, to write every day. Of course, I

have failed in all of these resolutions at one time or another. Overall, I'd give myself a B for the year.

All of this brings us back to an eternal question: what is the real self, who is my real self? I think it depends on the day, the mood, and the medication. About a year after we adopted Lyle, and maybe six months after in consultation with our vets we decided to put him on an antidepressant to control his separation anxiety and generalized frenetic behavior, I took him in for a checkup. Most vet techs I've met are women, usually young women who are hoping to become veterinarians. On this occasion several of the vet techs were walking through the waiting room together and noticed Lyle. They made a fuss over him, telling him how beautiful he was and so on, and he was on his best behavior. One said she had heard so many bad things about the numerous behavior problems of cocker spaniels that she had never considered having one, but one like Lyle could make her change her mind. Just as the techs were at their most gushing, Lyle's veterinarian, a sophisticated, witty, and young woman herself, walked by. Without a pause, she said, "*That* is a cocker spaniel on Prozac."

For almost an entire year now, I've been a human with cancer. Not just the chemo but simply having the disease changes you. In many ways, I think it can make you a better person if you are lucky enough to survive it, a better cocker spaniel, so to speak. The cancer has remade my self. I believe that the self is a narrative invention in the first place, so I don't believe that the cancer has uncovered my real self or my authentic self or my essential self. Those selves seem to me to be either the latest comfortable self or the latest most stable self. But one of the truisms of life, that experience makes or reveals what one really is, seems accurate to me. A physician might even point to me when I am being my best self and say, "*That* is a human being on cancer."

In some very strange way, having cancer can spoil you, at least if you survive your treatment and have a convincing remission.

For the many months I was in treatment, I felt, oddly, that I was the center of the universe. That can be a bad thing, of course, if you let it spoil you or if you take advantage of it, both results more difficult to avoid than you might think. You have an army of smart people, caring friends and relatives, nurses treating you with chemotherapy and even paying close attention to you because they know that helps your mood and therefore your possibility of survival. Then it's over with. You are in remission. And of course the question is "What do I do with the rest of my life now that I'm no longer the center of the universe and I'm no longer 'battling' for my life?" The deployment is over and it's time to go back home.

For me the final exit from chemotherapy brought on a month-long depression. That depression was deep enough to put me to sleep for ten hours a day and then to require a nap in the afternoon. It was probably partially because I felt that I wasn't fighting cancer anymore and wasn't the center of the universe, at least for that week out of each month. I'm still learning, I think, not to bring my cancer up in conversation unless it is relevant. For almost an entire year, cancer was the main topic of conversation and interest to me.

I'm looking forward to the day when I can take a three-hour bike ride with friends and not feel the necessity or urge to talk about cancer at all. That's when I won't be a cocker spaniel on Prozac. I'll be just a normal old dog (who can miraculously ride a bicycle). By the way, I fell today and landed on my helmet and felt my brain jostle inside my skull. So far, so good. No lasting injuries that I know of, although I did ask a friend a question about an hour after the fall that I had already asked and he had already answered that very day. Wear your helmets, my friends!

Heather Responds to
"On Not Being the Center of the Universe"

You may recall that a good friend of ours told me a month into his treatment, "It's not all about Don." I laughed but agreed, and Don said that he agreed as well when I told him (but his laugh wasn't very convincing). We've both shouldered burdens that we didn't think were possible a year ago. I think I have a pretty good sense of who I am. I'm never sure who Don is. He changes his preferences for diet, dress, music, and the company he keeps too quickly for me to pretend to keep up. His unpredictability is one of the things I like best about him. I'm looking forward to retirement not just because I'm tired of my job but because I have things that I want to do as well, such as volunteer for an organization that helps seniors and others with veterinary and pet food bills and expenses they can't afford. Many animals end up in shelters simply because their owners, through no fault of their own, can no longer afford to feed and care for them properly. I can't imagine a more heart-breaking experience than to have to give up my beloved pet to a shelter because I couldn't afford its medical bills.

Don will play guitars, read, write, and maybe publish, maybe fish. He talks about all of these things and about craving more time to do them. But who knows what will be next? One thing is sure: he will eventually find something that is not on his current list of activities and jump into that endeavor with the enthusiasm of a five-year-old with a new puppy.

I realize myself through reading, through reflection, and through interactions with others. Years of academic administration have almost ruined imaginative writing for me. I write brilliant proposals and legal documents and memos but could never write, for example, *Dear Committee Members*, a bitingly funny academic novel told through memos and letters.[1] It may be a long, long time before I can open my e-mail without flinching in anticipation of the next massively annoying thing that someone has done or said.

Don has said that he intends soon to no longer think of himself as "the guy with cancer." That is, of course, not likely in a literal sense. The thought may pass from being in his immediate consciousness on a daily basis. But we've been told that his cancer will likely return if he lives long enough. I think both of us have learned how to relegate this scary reality to a compartment in our minds, some place outside of the day-to-day but close enough that we can benefit from it. Even were the cancer not to return, I think Don will always be "with cancer" because the experience of it has changed his life. It has given him a new tenaciousness (like Cancer, the crab, itself) to accomplish his own personal goals. These are quite apart from his professional goals, which otherwise he might have been happy to pursue endlessly if cancer hadn't stepped in and said, "Hello, I'm here. Who knows? I might change your life for the better. It won't be easy." He writes of going to battle—but of course there's a difference between enlisting and simply finding bullets coming your way. Mortality affords lessons for the learning.

Notes

1. Schumacher, *Dear Committee Members.*

Afterward

September 16

YES, YOU READ THAT WORD CORRECTLY: *afterward,* not *after-word.* An afterword is usually the place to justify the writing of a book and perhaps also to thank the friends and colleagues who encouraged you in the writing along the way. I mean *afterward* to be understood as the adverb that it is, an opportunity to introduce what has happened since I was done with lymphoma. There's at least one more way that this "Afterward" is unlike an "Afterword." It's a long story.

I am still done with lymphoma, at least as long as I am in remission. But bad luck is not done with me, apparently. With one notable exception around New Year's, the fall and spring semesters after chemotherapy proceeded pretty much as I had expected, with slow and steady increase in strength and stamina. I stayed busy with teaching, committee work, and working on this book. Then I went to a national convention just after the New Year, unaware that a bout with pneumonia was brewing. The pneumonia was diagnosed after I visited an urgent care center in Austin. I spent most of the conference in bed taking antibiotics and resting. I had had a pneumonia vaccine for the first time that fall but, like a lot of other vaccines, it didn't guarantee that I wouldn't come down with pneumonia, especially if I ran myself ragged, as I did in the fall.

Heather retired in late December and stayed busy during much of the spring decompressing from her job and doing home projects she had put off while working.

After Heather's last day on the job in December, I told my department chair that I was intending to retire at the end of June. I doubt he was surprised. Early notice would give him and others in the department time to replace me with another linguist, if that's what the department needed, or with some other variety of English professor. Some folks upon retirement are heavily invested in who replaces them; me, I did not and do not have an opinion. Our English department is what is known in the business as a big tent department, meaning that we are friendly and open to all the varieties of what is practiced under the rubric of "English studies." It's a rare department that truly adheres to the big tent philosophy—UNR English does. It was a great place to work for eleven years. Throughout the spring semester I gradually moved all my books and knickknacks home from my office. I was expecting a quiet exit. I had told my friends that I didn't want a retirement party. No one raised a fuss. I'm not known for my partying ways.

Somewhere around the middle of April, four friends and Heather and I decided to check out a new Italian restaurant here in town. Three of the four friends drove over to our house and explained that the fourth would be busy for a few minutes more going over some paperwork at our department chair's house. Since his house was on the way to the restaurant, we would pick up our friend en route. The odd thing, though, was that one of my friends was shouting over his cell at the friend at the chair's house, and I could hear her shouting right back through the phone. Something alarming was going on, some kind of drama.

When we arrived at his house, my chair came out to the driveway and invited us in to see a new manuscript he had acquired (he collects them). In we walked, and there in his living room stood probably forty of my colleagues. My jaw went slack, and I looked around for the point of this gathering, but everybody was looking at me and grinning. I was the point. Somebody yelled, "Happy retirement!" and everyone clapped and cheered loudly. It felt for a moment sort of like I was an elementary school kid again and had walked into the wrong classroom. Once they were sure I wasn't going to seize up like an old tractor, one of my dearest friends led me to a closed guitar case.

"What's that?"

"It's yours, man. Open it!"

It was a brand-new Fender Telecaster. Which I was expected to *play* then and there because my friend had snuck in one of his own amplifiers. I was in too much shock to say no, so I bumbled through a Hendrix riff or two and hit the high E at the twelfth fret as my "solo," as I called it. But that wasn't all.

My manuscript-collecting chair had somehow procured a signed Christmas card that Flannery O'Connor, the writer I've spent a good part of my career writing about, had once sent to a friend. It felt humbling and strangely familiar to hold that framed card, which she had held once, adorned with her handwriting, which I instantly recognized: "We're still looking forward to that visit. Merry Christmas, Flannery."

I can't imagine the secret conspiring that it took to pull that surprise party off. I was gobsmacked, as the British say. As with my bicycle, I will probably never be worthy of the Telecaster, but it does encourage me to play every day and keep studying the guitar, on my list of retirement activities. It later came to light that the shouting over the phone was part of the ruse, the pretense of the unexpected necessity to stop by the chair's house. Or perhaps they were just having fun. Both shouting friends accused the other of overacting.

My department chair had spent days barbequing brisket, pork ribs, pork shoulder, and stuffed quail, plus preparing all the sides and dessert and everything else that comes with a big barbeque. They were all delicious, forcing me to revise my prejudice that you can barbeque brisket properly only if you are a native Texan. But I was able to sample only a small bit of each dish because all day I'd been experiencing abdominal cramping, due to what I didn't know. I figured it was attributable to nerves because I was approaching the end of the semester and then the pleasant shock of the party. I didn't think much about the cramping during the festivities since there were so many friends to talk with and hug and promise sincerely to stay in touch with.

The next day and night the cramps continued along with, and I hate to use this word, *constipation*. I dislike that word for many reasons, some of which I'll explain below, so instead I'll just use the word *concentration* and the verb that it is derived from, *concentrating*. You'll know what I mean, and I'll feel more comfortable. So it became apparent to me the next day that I was concentrating too hard. I'd had trouble with concentration before because of dehydration. So I just upped my water intake the next day and hoped to stop concentrating so damned hard. After all, I was headed to retirement in two weeks anyway, so it was time to start thinking about relaxing.

The second day after the party was a Sunday, and at about two in the morning I woke with intense pain in the upper right quadrant of my abdomen. Instead of trying to metaphorize the pain or try to describe it with a pile of adverbs, I'll just say this: I was unable to walk. I slowly crawled into the bathroom to look for Pepcid or anything that might relieve the pain. This is another aspect of human experience in which language fails us. How do you accurately and evocatively describe pain? The memory of the pain has faded now too, although not the memory of the terror. I swallowed some Pepcid and half a bottle of Tums, but nothing worked. My groaning woke Heather, who wanted to know what the hell I was doing writhing on the bathroom floor like a severed worm. I tried in vain to explain the pain, calling on an army of adjectives, adverbs, and metaphors (*very, intensely, sharp knives to my gut*). She called an EMT nurse hotline and described the symptoms. The nurse told Heather that her medical protocol computer program advised calling an ambulance immediately. The nurse ordered Heather to tell the EMTs to use "lights and sirens" to get me to the hospital because the symptoms could be indicative of lots of bad things like acute appendicitis or an aortic aneurysm. The ambulance was quick to arrive, and the EMTs were quick to relieve my pain with fentanyl, I believe it was.

The emergency room doctor ordered tests and scans to rule out aortic aneurysm and appendicitis. Later, both the doctor and the emergency room nurses found it amusing that I had such a bad case of concentration they couldn't even see my appendix on the CT scan. Ha ha.

To make a long, annoying story marginally less annoying, I'll cut to the chase and just say I was sent home with a prescription for Percocet and GOLYTELY, the latter frequently prescribed to patients in preparation for colonoscopies. I took the prescribed Percocet and dutifully eased my concentration the next day by drinking the gallon of GOLYTELY. It was a rough day, followed by an even harder night that was a rerun of the night before: the intense upper right abdominal pain recurred at 2:00 a.m., followed by another ambulance trip to the same emergency room, where I drew a different doctor and a different set of nurses and another CT. Before the CT could show that I was indeed not concentrating anymore, I was given a completely unnecessary industrial-strength enema—another word I hate—and sent home without pain medication because I already had a prescription that I hadn't finished. The nurse who administered the enema seemed terribly excited about the procedure, I think because he had never administered such a powerful, I would say even mother of all enemas before. He called it a Pink Lady. Because there was almost nothing in my bowels, which the results of the CT scan clearly showed later, the results of the enema were pathetic compared to the almost military might of the enema itself. When I came back to the treatment room from the bathroom, the nurse had disappeared.

I never saw him again. He had launched the enema and abandoned the territory, I guess assuming that he had hit his target. In truth there was no target to hit, but the treatment room did look like a bloodless battlefield. The hoses and container for the enema were left on the floor as well as once-sterile gloves and protective drapes. I lay back on the table, pushing the remainder of the detritus to the floor, and waited despondently to be fetched by Heather or yet another nurse.

The third night, earlier in the evening the pain returned, along with a new one: burning pain in the lower back. The pain in my abdomen and my back were barely distinguishable. They merged into a greater pain than I'd experienced the first two nights. Heather talked by phone with a charge nurse, whose judgment was that I probably shouldn't have been sent home the second night without a surgical consultation. I decided to try another emergency room in town because I was concerned that the first simply assumed that the problem must have been the concentration, but that had been eliminated, so to speak.

The mistake I made with the third trip to the different ER, a mistake that I will never, ever make again, was that I didn't ride in an ambulance because it had been so embarrassing riding with the same EMTs two nights in a row. Instead, a friend drove Heather and me. What I didn't know is that if you don't arrive by ambulance you are not seen right away but instead are triaged and usually have to wait for treatment behind others who might or might not have more serious ailments—but some got there by ambulance. Not that I could tell how many were in the waiting room ahead of me or how many might have more serious medical emergencies than I did because after shuffling in with my head hung down, making eye contact only with the floor, I found myself on the floor on my knees with my head in my hands writhing in an empty chair. All I heard was a patient apparently having some kind of psychotic episode because she kept yelling, "She's looking at me!" repeatedly and at ever-increasing volume.

I was eventually wheeled back to an emergency room bed, where a diligent doctor inserted an IV himself to get pain medication into me as soon as possible. He examined my abdomen and back carefully and said, "I'm not sure, but your pain in the back may be the early onset of shingles before the rash." I had no idea I was even at risk for shingles because I had received the shingles vaccination years before and considered myself safe. The ER doctor explained that the vaccination does not guarantee that one will not get shingles, but that if one does, usually the case is milder than it would have been otherwise. Just like the pneumonia. He said that he would prescribe a stronger dose of oxycodone and an anti-viral and advised me to see my family physician as soon as possible. He told us that a nurse would be in soon with the written prescription. I supposed that he didn't have his pad with him at the time or that the prescription had to be recorded in the hospital's computer system.

After the doctor left the room, I went to the bathroom to pee. On my way back, I saw one of the nurses on duty who had first helped attend to me sitting at a computer terminal. He hadn't talked to me; the ER physician had asked and answered all questions thus far. We made eye contact. I smiled. He smirked and rolled his eyes. I was clueless about how to react to that other than to go into immediate denial because that's my normal response to social aggression of that sort: "I simply can't have seen what I think I just saw. He has no reason to despise me, although that seems to be clearly indicated by his face and actions." I went back to the emergency room bed and Heather and thought nothing more of it for the time being. I was simply longing for a good long sleep and an appointment with my family physician soon to get this mystery sorted out. We waited another fifteen minutes and then Heather, rightly worrying that we were probably taking up space that was needed for the next patient in the triage line, went to the nurse's station to ask the nurse whether he had the doctor's prescription for the stronger oxycodone. The nurse gave

Heather the prescription and came back to the room with her; I wasn't sure why. Heather asked the nurse when I could next take the pain medication because I had just had an IV dose. That's when the nurse started yelling angrily, "He shouldn't take *any* for at least eight hours. I've seen his records, and his problem is that he is constipated [no, in fact I wasn't concentrating anymore, as the scan of the previous night had shown], and the narcotics only make it worse! He's on a spiral, first one emergency room visit and then another, shopping for narcotics!" This rant woke me up to what his malfunction was. I got within an inch of his nose and yelled right back, "I am *not* a drug addict, and I am *not* constipated [concentrating]. What the *hell* is *wrong* with you?!" He had no answer, just stomped out of the room, leaving us to pick up our belongings and leave.

As I briefly mentioned early in this book, just since I've been writing here about my shoulder surgeries and experiences with oxycodone, the United States has been hit with what appears to be an epidemic of prescription painkiller abuse, among both celebrities and garden-variety humans. A recent *Harper's* "Index" reports that three-fifths "of Americans prescribed painkillers in the past year . . . have leftovers in their home," and one-fifth "have shared them with someone else."[1] I do have leftovers from prescriptions given even later this summer, locked away in a very secure gun safe, but I have never and would never share them with someone. In fact, what I will probably do is what I've done before: take them to my regular pharmacy and ask staff to dispose of them safely. I realize that this epidemic of abuse of prescription narcotics is disturbing, but to use an admittedly poor analogy, just because some poor souls sniff paint or glue, we don't normally yell at people in hardware stores as they are buying paint or glue for home repair. The epidemic is so serious and widespread that when Heather and I went to a local pharmacy at 6:00 a.m. to fill the prescription for the stronger oxycodone, a very polite self-described homeless man chatted with Heather and then attempted to buy some of the oxycodone from her. He said he "doesn't need it but really likes oxycodone," Heather reported. I didn't witness the conversation because by that time the emergency room painkillers had begun to wear off and I was pacing the aisles of the drugstore, breathing deeply but slowly, trying not to start moaning again. The pharmacist told Heather that what I was given at the emergency room was fast acting and fast disappearing and that I could start taking the oxycodone in another thirty minutes as long as I stuck to the schedule, which I always do.

I've never abused the painkillers I've been prescribed, and I've never taken more than the dose prescribed by either a surgeon or a pain specialist. In fact, if I've made any mistake with them at all, it has been in trying too hard to do without them. As many health-care professionals will tell you, staying ahead of the pain is always easier than playing catch up. I do feel deeply for anyone who loses their life or a loved one to addiction, whether it's opiates, alcohol, or tobacco. Two of my friends have died from the horrible physical effects of alcoholism. One I knew was an alcoholic; I hadn't a single suspicion about the other. I never thought he had more than a beer or two at most with friends on any given day. I thought I knew him well.

At this point, just after the pharmacist has filled the latest prescription for pain medication, Heather and I have had about two hours of sleep per night for three nights in a row. So now we sleep most of the middle of the day away, but then I wake up at about 3:00 p.m.: the pain is back, uncontrolled by the prescribed dosage of oxycodone. Since it is Monday, Heather calls to see whether she can get me in to see my family physician, who has been out of town but makes room for me in his schedule for Tuesday morning after hearing the story of the last three nights. Somehow I make it through the night by pacing, sleeping, watching movies, and taking the pain medication when prescribed. Lyle sleeps with Heather that night.

My family physician looks over my back (no rash yet) and

palpates my abdomen, murmuring that the pain suggests appendicitis but that the labs and scans don't show it. He apologizes for what he has to do next, "just to be sure," since pain in the abdomen can be referred from many places. He palpates my prostate, which doesn't hurt as much as it normally does given all the other competing pain. He finds nothing conclusive but says I need to be admitted to the hospital for a surgical consult. He will call ahead to order the admission. Heather suggests that I take an ambulance from his office, which I do.

The doctor at the hospital, a new one to me, is as puzzled as everyone else and says, "I hate to ask you this, but this pain you are having can be referred from almost anywhere. Do you mind if I palpate your testicles?" I shrug. "Why not? My family doctor just had his finger up my ass thirty minutes ago."

It winds up taking almost twenty-four hours to get a surgical consult. I'm kept in a pre-op room and medicated heavily. Once the surgeon (whom I do not know) examines me, he tells Heather that I'm in so much pain they should probably observe me for another day. Because he hasn't had time to examine my history, Heather informs him that this is my fourth emergency room visit for pain in as many days. He says, "Oh, my rule is three strikes and you're out." And he trots off to schedule an operating room within thirty minutes.

After surgery, the surgeon tells Heather that it turns out on laparoscopically examining my abdomen that I had a Meckel's diverticulum, an embryonic intestinal malformation that 2 percent of the world's population has. Of that 2 percent, only somewhere between 2 percent to 5 percent have any difficulty in their lifetime, and the majority of those have the problem before the age of two. Unresolved childhood intestinal issues. The Meckel's diverticulum, really just a pouch that hangs off the ileum portion of the small intestine, is the remnant of the embryonic yolk sac. It should have atrophied and been absorbed by my embryonic self by seven weeks' gestation. Perhaps I was distracted. Common symptoms of a Meckel's diverticulum include abdominal pain and intense concentration.[2]

My new surgeon snipped off the diverticulum, the grotesqueness of which you may or may not want to think about or google. For good measure, he also took my appendix, which was fine, thanks very much, but which is known to be a frequent trouble maker so good riddance. And then there was the recovery, which was almost as bad as the disease since if you disturb your guts they tend to "shut down" and their electrical system goes haywire, which can sometimes be permanent.

Spoiler alert: before this drama was over, I had to have two abdominal surgeries. This first one, laparoscopic, and another that was open abdominal. None of my previous surgeries—for shoulder or lymph biopsies—seemed as invasive as either of the abdominal surgeries, even the first laparoscopic one. There is something intensely personal about abdominal surgery, as if your very essence is being disturbed—cut, severed, partially removed, invaded. Both psychologically and physically, the pain feels located at one's core being. If you care to peer down the rabbit hole of just Western (as opposed to the vast Eastern literature as well) labyrinthine understandings of the location(s) of the soul, a traditional place to begin is Plato, who in some interpretations located only one part of a three-part soul in the abdomen.[3] I'm sure that if I'd had heart surgery or neurosurgery, I would have felt my essential soul being jostled and prodded and poked somewhere in my chest or between my two ears. Contemporary scientists are also hard at work in the study of the two-way communication pathways between our brains and our alimentary canal (our digestive system, which scientists sometimes refer to as our "second brain").[4]

After the first abdominal surgery, I had to stay on the post-surgical floor until I was almost batty with lack of sleep and the stress of sharing a hospital room with a dead ringer, in appearance, voice, and personality, for Buffalo Bill in *Silence of the Lambs*. My roommate played his television (we both had one) with the volume on high even when he was snoring like a drunk nineteenth-century miner. His wife apparently disliked me because she mistook a nurse's information that everyone had earphones for their TV as an indication that I had complained about the noise of Buffalo Bill's TV. She angrily and loudly told the nurse, "Our TV is not too loud, and he has his own if he wants to watch something else." I could not even imagine the noise of the Kardashians competing with the noise of whatever I would choose, likely *The Three Stooges* if I could find them. I in fact hadn't complained about the noise, but by the time I felt it was appropriate to complain the tension in the hospital room was thick.

Later in my first day on the post-surgical floor, Bill's daughter, who was pre-med (he told me), came to visit him for the first time, although he had already been in the hospital for four days and was in at least as much pain as I was.

B. BILL: So, what you been up to?

PRE-MED DAUGHTER (*sucking a 32-ounce soda through double-barreled straws*): Oh, nothing much, just hanging out at John's.

B. BILL: Oh.

PRE-MED DAUGHTER: Dad, you're so *old*.

B. BILL: *You're* old!

PRE-MED DAUGHTER: You could have just died.

B. BILL: Yeah.

(*Awkward silence, filled by raucous laughter from reality TV*)

PRE-MED DAUGHTER: Well, I better go.

B. BILL: Okay, your mom will be back up later.

PRE-MED DAUGHTER: Okay, bye.

By the next day in recovery, I was electively mute. During Heather's visit on the second day, I couldn't answer any of her questions other than by nodding or shaking my head or shrugging my shoulders. She was visibly alarmed at my mental turn for the worse. I honestly don't know why I had gone mute: trauma, pain, I don't know.

I think part of my worry resulted from a faux pas I had committed earlier that day. To get to the toilet in my room, I had to cross the barrier between my side of the room and B. Bill's. B. Bill normally had visitors, loud visitors, and I was ashamed of having to go the toilet so frequently and often so unsuccessfully to check whether my bowels had started working again. So even though the nurses had told me not to use the public restrooms, of which there were four in the long hallways of the surgical recovery floor, I used them anyway, twice. I walked around the hallways quite a bit, which both the nurses and my surgeon encouraged. I had little strength as yet, so I mostly held on to the top of my IV tree, pushing or pulling it on my travels. I was on heavy painkillers during the two days following surgery, so I was kind of groggy walking around, although it was certainly preferable to lying in that noisy, dark hospital room.

In walking the floor, I saw other patients out walking like myself, either by themselves or with what were probably friends or family. One grandfatherly figure, dressed in hospital chic like I was, hospital gown and slip-resistant socks, appeared to be walking with his granddaughter, who looked maybe seventeen or eighteen. There are social norms to obey in the hallway: no staring, for one. You can notice other people, but don't stare. People come and go in the hallway. When I came out of the bathroom the second time, I was especially woozy, my eyes slowly coming into focus as I stood outside the bathroom adjusting the lines to my various IV drips, making sure that nothing was tangled. Once I got my eyes focused, I looked up to see the girl I had noticed earlier with her grandfather staring at me in bug-eyed horror. Before I could react, she turned away in an almost military about-face and walked off quickly toward the elevators down another hallway. What the hell? Then I looked down and brought my eyes to focus on my clothing. One side of my hospital gown was hiked up and tucked inside my boxer shorts, half of which were showing— along with my spindly old man's legs. I was horrified. I went back to the room, slipped into bed, stuffed earplugs deep into my ear canals, and tried not to think the words *trauma, indecent exposure,* or *probation*. I hadn't really exposed anything obscene, but never- theless, as the young say, "Some things cannot be unseen." Like my plaid boxers, for instance. When, three weeks later, I could finally bring myself to tell the story to a female friend, she said the inci- dent showed one thing clearly: I do *not* know how to wear a dress.

After about three days in post-op, my guts self-jump-started and I was fine except for the pain from the three incisions. I was released from the hospital with strict instructions not to lift any- thing heavy. I insisted on teaching one final class of one of my courses to finish out the semester. Heather was my guardian so that I wouldn't do something really stupid, besides teach the class in the first place. Heather proctored one final exam for me, and a colleague did the same for the other. So things seemed almost back to normal.

My surgeon, Heather tells me, sent my Meckel's diverticu- lum off for a biopsy. Back at home, I slowly recovered, with lots of post-operative pain, probably because of the bonus of the shin- gles, which would take three weeks to clear completely. I received an e-mail from the hospital a few days after my release saying that my pathology report was ready to view online. I hadn't seen my surgeon or my oncologist since being released because they were both on what I was sure were well-deserved vacations. I didn't read the path report right away because I expected it to essen- tially say nothing. But then, like a dumbass, I read it late one night, about eleven. The report said that there was a carcinoid tumor in the Meckel's diverticulum, and that it was impossible to tell whether the surgeon got it all because it grew up to the staple line from where it was separated from my ileum. The report starkly stated that there were cancer cells present at the staple site and in the lymph vesicle leading away from site. Both NIH and Merck websites report that carcinoid tumors in Meckel's diverticula are not uncommon.[5]

I couldn't catch my breath. Every time I tried to inhale, it was as if my lungs were already full of air. I was having one of my familiar panic attacks, although I wouldn't have been able to name it so at the time. Cancer! Again! An unrelated cancer! In my intestines! Crying, I woke Heather up and told her about the path report. She explained that the surgeon had told her after the operation that he was suspicious of the tissue but that he couldn't tell for certain whether it was cancerous. Heather hadn't told me earlier so that I wouldn't worry unnecessarily. My wife has a will of iron. There is no way I could have kept such a secret for close to a week. What she didn't expect was that the hospital would send me the pathology report before either the surgeon or my oncologist had had time to speak with me about it. And she certainly didn't expect that I would be dumb enough to look at it at 11:00 p.m.

I saw the surgeon a few days later. He wanted to go back into surgery that week or the next (unless I was, say, "going to Paris for a once-in-a-lifetime trip") and take out eight inches of my small intestine, plus surrounding tissue and lymph nodes, to be sure he got it all, to be sure that he had clean margins. But even that, he said, wouldn't guarantee that there weren't cancer cells hiding elsewhere. He estimated five to ten days of recovery in the hospital from this second surgery since it couldn't be done laparoscopically. He said it would hurt worse than the last time but that I would have a morphine pump this time. He called my oncologist for a consult. My oncologist wanted me to undergo octreotide scans first to determine whether and how far the carcinoids had spread. Good idea, that. I tried to console myself with the knowledge that it could turn out to be nothing. True, or it could turn out to be the worst news possible.

This was the time for all that philosophical reading and big-picture-taking on life to kick in.

Three days of intense scanning started June 6. The good news was that if more surgery was necessary, the wait would give me more time to recover, especially since the subsequent surgery promised to be more disruptive to my normal goodwill toward life than the first surgery. My hope was that the very thorough scanning would show nothing and that surgery would not be necessary then (which was at least a remote possibility, I mistakenly thought). The only downside was that if I did have metastasized abdominal carcinoids, the wait might give the bastards time to cause more trouble.

The goal of the scanning technicians over three days was to make an entire three-dimensional map of the interior of my body, with the hopes that if I had carcinoids elsewhere they would show up like glittering gold in the slush of my intestines and organs. Thus, the surgeon would know more precisely where to stab me. The morning of the first day of scanning, I was injected with radioactive octreotide and told to stay away from children and pregnant women because I would be "hot." The octreotide is attracted to receptors on the carcinoids, so whatever is not attached to them gets flushed, I'm sure right down the river, to be scrubbed ineffectively for drinking water later. I was ordered to come back four hours later, at which point I was wrapped in a warm blanket and placed under the largest camera lens I've ever seen, which also traveled the length of my body. A lens underneath was filming my bum as well. I call them lenses because, even though they detect radioactivity, I imagined them to be large blind eyes, with industrial beige plastic covering them. I think I entered a Zen state. I was told that I could eat nothing, essentially, but broth for the next two days. It took a total of three days to get a complete map of my innards.

And . . . the scans showed nothing. They were negative.

My oncologist and surgeon both broke the bad news to me that I would have to undergo surgery anyway. So the official story going into surgery was that there was no metastasis and that even though this would be an open rather than a laparoscopic surgery, the surgeon would simply be trying to ensure that he had clean margins on either side of the incision that marked the place where my diverticulum was. I had prepared a joke for the operating room:

ME: Knock-knock.

SURGEON: Who's there?

ME: Bond.

SURGEON: Bond who?

ME: Don Bond . . . Har, har, har! . . . I'm high!

Heather stopped responding to "knock-knock" by three days before the scheduled surgery. I think she was looking forward to some peace and quiet during my five to ten days on the ward.

I told several of my friends that I doubted I would be very good company during the days I would be in the hospital, but since I would be under the influence of morphine for much of the time, there would be a pretty good chance that I could be persuaded to speak in tongues.

In the two days leading up to the surgery, I ate nothing but frozen yogurt and liquids of various sorts all day long. I didn't want any unpleasant surprises in the OR. I was planning to flirt shamelessly with my anesthesiologist. My uneducated opinion is that in the OR the anesthesiologist is the only one who stands a serious chance of either killing you or making you very, very happy for a relatively short period of time. I was aiming for the latter.

My surgeon was able to get me a single occupancy room, for which I was and am enormously grateful. I did not want to run into B. Bill again. The most exciting thing about what turned out to be the surprisingly short five-day hospital stay for recovery was the time someone set my morphine drip alarm to go off when the supply was completely gone. That alarm is supposed to go off an hour before the morphine will run dry. So I ran dry suddenly at maybe three in the afternoon. And the thing about morphine is that it acts quickly—and stops acting even more quickly. I was like a skinned cat holding on by my claws to the ceiling. At the time, I thought yet again that it was a good thing I was in a single room. I can't imagine how upsetting a roommate would have found it to have me screaming in pain and four or five nurses scrambling trying to figure out what went wrong and how to fix it.

I did a lot of walking, but I always wore a bathrobe over my gown to guarantee there would be no more accidental traumatic exposures.

A follow-up appointment with my surgeon revealed that the carcinoids had in fact already metastasized despite not showing up on the scan. Heather already knew this. The surgeon had told her immediately after the surgery while I was still in recovery. The surgeon was able to remove two carcinoids while he was in, but there was at least one other that he wasn't able to get to. The mystery is, obviously, why the three days of nuclear scans didn't find the other carcinoids. Internet research showed me that treatment possibilities included hormones (the main option), radiation, or—more chemo.

I saw my oncologist about a week after being released from the hospital. He said he would consult with a gastroenterologist and carcinoid specialist at Stanford and then talk with me again in three weeks. He mentioned everything from watch and wait (which is now again the situation with the lymphoma) to hormone therapy (of what ungodly sort I don't know) to experimental treatment in San Francisco. At this point, I was sick of the whole damn thing. And my onc wanted to talk about it *again* in three weeks.

So they're still there, the carcinoids, with possible metastasizing landing sites being other spots on ileum, liver, or pancreas. The *good* thing about carcinoids is that they are supposed to be very slow to grow, and the surgeon did accidentally find mine early because he had to remove the diverticulum. This living in death's shadow shit is hard to talk about because everyone is in

raining his new nurse how to
perform the procedure), he said it would feel like bee stings. These
guys really need to work on their similes. In actuality, it was closer
to "like having staples pulled out of your abdomen." But that's
done, and the onc called back soon and said the Stanford specialist
in carcinoids believes there's nothing really to do for my carcinoid
infestation (my term) at this stage except an octreotide scan every
six months (not sure how much I trust that method) and special
tests of urine and blood every three months. The only thing about
this that's mildly interesting is that the urine test requires collect-
ing urine for twenty-four hours straight. I'm going to treat this
part like a competition with myself. How much piss can I deliver
to the lab every three months? I'm guessing they will need less
blood.

ponds to
"Afterward"

As you can imagine after reading "Afterward," late spring and
summer were awful. While dealing with the ordeal of Don's surgeries, I was also dealing with my cat Lamar's multiple surgeries
for mast cell tumors, skin cancers that required him to undergo
biopsies and then resections. The worst part for him was that he
had to wear dog T-shirts to keep him from pulling out his stitches.
He's a better patient than Don, resignedly tolerating all the surgeries under local anesthesia. On the other hand, Don never gnawed
out his stitches. I felt like I had no role other than medic and care-
giver during this period.

I needed a break. Badly. Once he had recovered from the surgeries, Don was writing nonstop. So I took a trip to Idaho to a resort lake with a friend while Don stayed in Reno looking after the house and the animals. He had had his break the previous week in northeastern California, mostly alone working on this book at a cabin in a cell phone and Internet dead zone. Don got this opportunity to play Thoreau because one of his friends was teaching several days at a writers' workshop in a nearby town. He called the experience bliss. He said he saw several mule deer and lizards. The area featured a playa and some mountains. Don had a long talk with the woman who comes to water the plants and orchard behind and around the cabin when the owners are not there. They bonded over how nice it is to live a mile from your nearest neighbor. Don's been sending me web page after web page of available real estate in the neighborhood of this playa. Dream on.

Anyway, he wanted me to write this response while I was on my own vacation. Not my idea of a good time, writing about ordeals and cancer and so on. I have just a few observations to make. I can't understand how Don could possibly fail to mention the submarine sandwich. It was one of the only humorous parts of the many ER visits. You might imagine that the answer lies in his squeamishness about constipation. Really. Having to use a euphemism like *concentration*. It's like Mary Roach after first mention proceeding to call *maggots* by the euphemism (I guess) *haciendas* in one of her many fine books on topics that others find gross.[6] At least that made me laugh out loud. *Concentration* seems precious in comparison, but it explains why Don left the sandwich discussion to me. What happened was that a youngish ER doc waltzed in with a grin on his face and described the image he had just seen on the CT scan as "a poop ball the size of a submarine sandwich," demonstrating its size with his hands in the air. Don didn't find this funny. And didn't when I repeated it frequently thereafter. And still doesn't. In fact he has often referred to this event, borrowing the response of a friend of his to the story, as "the final gasping dying breath of what was left of [my] already frayed dignity."

One thing we've discovered after all of this is that he can't remember a lot of what happened when he was in the hospital, and he's often inaccurate in what he can recall. Understandable, given the pain and the medication. For instance, he didn't learn that the surgery wasn't curative (surgeon's word) from the surgeon later on, but from me as soon as they wheeled him into his hospital room after the procedure. The surgeon told me, leaving it to me to inform Don. I remember well because as I sat for four hours waiting to see him while they found him a post-op bed, the whole time I was trying to think how best to tell him, still trying to absorb the news and its implications myself. He took the news very well, actually commenting idly that maybe his calm reaction was because of the morphine. He has continued to handle it well, although he had his moments of terror that he told me about only much later, like the deep feelings of invasiveness the abdominal surgeries evoked.

I have a theory. I think that once you have had to confront intensely that truth of your own mortal self, the fear and uncertainty that entails, and the fact of having incurable cancer (even if in a world with new therapeutic breakthroughs almost daily), a second diagnosis is somehow less terrifying. Or perhaps simply tiresome, as he hints in this chapter. Being whipsawed between hope and dread is more bearable the second time around, and perhaps the consolation of philosophy is easier to find, as Don's musings on the self suggest. Me, I find Sam Harris's views on the self in *Waking Up* comforting.[7] To simplify a beautiful, erudite argument, and at the risk of sounding like *The Matrix*: there is no self. If we can find a way to believe that, we have found the path to bliss.

Notes

1. "Index," 9.
2. Burke, "Meckel's Diverticulum."

3. Plato, *The Republic of Plato*, 129-38.

4. Hadhazy, "Think Twice."

5. Rabinowitz, "Pediatric Meckel Diverticulum"; Baum and Companioni, "Meckel Diverticulum"; Dumper et al., "Complications of Meckel's Diverticula in Adults."

6. Roach, *Stiff*, 65.

7. Harris, *Waking Up*, 86-89.

Research Interlude

October 14

IN A KIND OF METAPHORICAL SENSE, unless you are a cancer researcher yourself, everything you know about cancer is part of the history of cancer because the methods of cancer treatment, or even who owns a cancer therapy, change so rapidly. In the spring of 2015, when I was recovering from chemotherapy and getting my life back in order, a company named AbbVie Inc. acquired ibrutinib, by the brand name of Imbruvica, from Pharmacyclics LLC. AbbVie paid $21 billion to acquire Pharmacyclics, "getting the rights of blockbuster molecule, Imbruvica."[1] *Forbes* reports that Pharmacyclics' former CEO Robert Duggan "earned $3.5 billion in cash and stock from the deal before taxes." *Forbes* estimates Duggan's net worth at $2.6 billion as of September 19, 2016.[2]

In 2013, the cost of ibrutinib for CLL was estimated at $98,400 per year, as I mentioned earlier.[3] After AbbVie's acquisition, the *Wall Street Journal* reported in December 2015, Imbruvica's "whole-sale list price" had risen to "$116,600 a year for leukemia patients" and the cost of "the higher dose needed for lymphoma" came in at "about $155,400" a year. As Joseph Walker points out in the article, companies that produce high-dollar drugs frequently offer discount coupons, but sometimes patients with insurance or Medicare are still too strapped to cover the cost of the co-pay for the medication. Some patients in the middle class "make too much money to qualify for assistance. Others are unaware the programs exist. Medicare patients, who represent nearly a third of

U.S. retail drug spending, can't receive direct aid from drug companies."[4] The result is that sometimes people who need this medication simply cannot afford it. Walker notes, "AbbVie declined to comment on the drug's price." Because my CLL/SLL was manifested most obviously in grotesquely swelling lymph nodes, I'm guessing I will need the higher, more expensive dose if I fail remission and no other effective treatments are available.

Bruce Cheson, MD in the Division of Hematology/Oncology at Georgetown University and the Lombardi Comprehensive Cancer Center, says ibrutinib (Imbruvica) is now approved as the treatment of first choice for two types of CLL patients: (1) those who have the 17p deletion, and (2) those too frail to withstand chemotherapy. It can also be an option for those who don't fall into those categories. Jason M. Broderick reports, "When discussing ibrutinib versus chemotherapy options with patients, Cheson covers delivery method (oral ibrutinib vs IV chemotherapy), toxicity (usually higher with chemotherapy), and length of treatment ('indefinitely' with ibrutinib versus '6 months and done' with chemotherapy)."[5] There is no word from Broderick in his article about whether Cheson discusses market forces with his patients.

Never fear, though. Duggan put everything in context: paraphrasing Duggan, Joseph Walker writes, "The price represents [Imbruvica's] value in the marketplace. After patents expire in about 15 years, a generic version will be much cheaper." Walker then quotes Duggan: "'That's where society wins. People look at it in the very short term.'"[6]

Well, I have short-term goals myself. I'm currently sixty-one years old. I'd like to live to, perhaps, at least seventy-six. So, let's say that AbbVie's patent expires in my seventy-sixth year, that is, that its patent extends from 2016 to 2030. That would mean that if my FCR remission fails sometime this year and I have to go on Imbruvica and it works for me, say, *short term* for fifteen years, I and my insurance company will pay AbbVie approximately $2.3 million (wholesale)—an estimate that assumes the price of

Imbruvica does not rise a dollar in those fifteen years. To assume a rather extreme fictional world, if I had, say, $2.5 billion, I could buy Imbruvica for myself, wholesale, for 16,087½ years with no insurance coverage at all. Or that same $2.5 billion could pay the wholesale cost for one year's treatment of Imbruvica for 16,087½ people afflicted with lymphoma. The National Cancer Institute estimates 20,110 new cases of CLL in 2017. The estimated number of deaths from CLL in 2017 is 4,660.[7] These figures kind of make $2.5 billion sound like a lot of money for one individual or not that much money at all (in fact, wholly inadequate) for the aggregate of Americans newly diagnosed with CLL each year.

Oh, and think fast because there is another CLL drug with great promise in line to be serious competition for Imbruvica. It goes by the name of acalabrutinib and is owned by a different company, Acerta Pharma, whose majority equity stake is held by AstraZeneca.[8] I cannot wait to follow the investment and pricing dramas surrounding the competition of Imbruvica and acalabrutinib if the latter lives up to its early promise to perhaps outperform Imbruvica in keeping people like me alive with perhaps fewer negative side effects. It's what I do instead of playing fantasy football. It's like fantasy football in that I can have no real effect on the outcome, yet I can't help but think that all those multibillion-dollar investors are thinking of me when they deliver a bone-crunching counteroffer in a pharmaceutical corporate takeover.

After reading this chapter, Heather said that she would be glad when I turned my research skills to home repair, lawn maintenance, or "showing a certain cocker spaniel that he's not the boss of me."

Heather Responds to
"Research Interlude"

Originally, I wasn't going to respond to Don's factual and obsessively numerical account of the cost of cancer drugs and pharmaceutical company profits. However, I've spent countless hours of late signing up for Medicare and comparing supplemental insurance plans, including those for prescription drug coverage (Part D). As a retiree under sixty-five, Don continues on our employer's plan, and out-of-pocket costs are capped at $3,900. At sixty-five, retirees have to go on Medicare and then enter the state exchange for supplemental insurance. From what I can tell, even for me drug costs are going to be much higher than before, even under the best plans. We are no different from the millions of other Americans struggling with drug costs that are taking up higher and higher percentages of their income and savings. And when you're laboring under the strain of a life-threatening illness, the threat of bankruptcy or an uncertain financial future is too much.

The American Association of Retired Persons (AARP) is one of the major lobbyists on behalf of older Americans, and one of their top concerns of late has been the increasingly high cost of prescription drugs. The cover story of a recent issue of the *AARP Bulletin* focuses on the causes of these costs and what consumers can do about them. In their discussion of the costs of bringing drugs to market, the editors point out that pharmaceutical company profit margins compare quite favorably to some of the other "successful and well-known American companies, for 2016," showing AbbVie at number two (below Amgen) and AstraZeneca at number nine (below Verizon); the percentages were 36.6 percent and 21.3 percent, respectively. Thanks to highly effective (and pricey) lobbying of legislators by pharmaceutical companies, Medicare cannot even negotiate drug prices.[9] It remains to be seen whether increasing pressure from the public will result in successful legislative efforts in Congress or the states. Of course, those who believe that the open market should determine everything will oppose government negotiation as "price control." And as Don pointed out, Medicare recipients are not eligible for the "discounting" that some pharmaceutical companies offer to offset costs and cost increases.

I take this personally.

Notes

1. "AbbVie Inc Imbruvica, Magical Molecule for Rare Disease."
2. "Robert Duggan."
3. Corner, "Ibrutinib's Breakthrough to Market."
4. Walker, "Patients Struggle with High Drug Prices."
5. Broderick, "Cheson Highlights Choices in Frontline CLL Care."
6. Walker, "Patients Struggle with High Drug Prices."
7. "Cancer Stat Fact Sheets: Chronic Lymphocytic Leukemia (CLL)."
8. Shaffer, "Next-Generation BTK Inhibitor Taking on Ibrutinib in CLL"; "AstraZeneca Completes Transaction for Majority Equity Stake Investment in Acerta Pharma."
9. Editors of AARP, "Why Drugs Cost So Much," 18.

Epilogue

November 2016

HOW DO YOU WRITE a last chapter to a book like this without getting all tangled up in the worst clichés imaginable? I trust your imagination, but if you need some help, here are a few: "I appreciate life more; every day, every minute now counts; I don't hold grudges; I never get angry or depressed; I tell my wife that I love her every day, and I don't just tell her, I act on it—roses (actually, she finds them 'boring'), candy (she hates it), breakfast in bed (I almost never get up first)." So much for romantic clichés. I know that I do appreciate Heather more now, although I struggle with ways to manifest that love and appreciation. I also appreciate more than I did before all the friends who helped us through the ordeals, although it's possible to overdo thanks there as well. I never know whether I've underdone it or overdone it. Cancer is not a magic bullet for our disorderly selves.

I've been imagining how to avoid the clichés that an epilogue almost invites: I might narrate an imaginary noir ending of walking to the local deli for some milk for my coffee, looking the wrong way, and getting hammered by a speeding recycling truck. I know I've seen this scene in a number of movies that didn't seem to know quite how to end themselves. It's respectable, but it would give the lie to the foolishly optimistic promise, which I recognized on rereading but decided to leave in, that this book would not end like all dog books. Who am I to promise not to die before the book is finished? Pretty much shows that I haven't learned as much as I'd like to think.

Or, since I'm just now getting around to reading Bram Stoker's *Dracula,* I thought maybe I'd philosophize about the dead undead, blood, and our current book, TV, and movie obsession with varieties of the dead undead.

I asked a good friend what she thought I should do with this last chapter. She's about forty years younger than I am, so honestly I thought I'd just throw out the problem and see how she hit the ball back. Without hesitation, she said I should write about how other people think I've changed in reaction to the cancers.

I thought, "Perfect. This will give all my friends an excuse to wax on and on about how much kinder and thoughtful and mindful I've become." So I was going to interview a few folks, not give their names, probably fictionalize most of what they say, and call it done.

I naturally first asked my friend who had come up with the suggestion. She said, "You didn't used to talk about blood and pee so much...I mean, it's interesting, but I never thought I'd find it interesting." In truth, I rarely have the opportunity to bubble with enthusiasm about the search for too much serotonin in my blood or a metabolite of serotonin (5-HIAA) in my urine every three months, as oncologists search for signs of my intestinal carcinoids becoming overactive.[1] But my friend was kind to listen to me and at least pretend that she found it interesting. I don't know. I imagine my obsessions with serotonin and 5-HIAA will fade into the background, just as I don't now think daily about my white blood cells.

My next interviewee was Heather:

ME: How do you think the cancers have changed me?

HEATHER: Never mind about that. I'm just wondering about you, like I've wondered about all the fucking men in my life, whether you ever worry about what I'm thinking. Like maybe how the cancers have changed *me*.

ME: What?

HEATHER: Do you ever worry or even wonder about what I'm thinking?

ME: No, because you are constantly telling me what you're thinking. But I do wonder now why you lumped me in with all the "fucking men" in your life.

HEATHER: I said that just to see if I'd get a reaction.

ME: See what I mean?

HEATHER: No.

So much for the interviews. I decided to spare my remaining friends and family. Heather did tell me yesterday that it isn't Lyle that has separation anxiety. It's me. I worry when he's in the backyard. I worry about him getting out and coyotes or bears getting him. They come around occasionally in our city. A befuddled mountain lion tried to walk into a casino a couple of years back. Although news of my separation anxiety came as a surprise to me and although I still believe that Lyle is the one who has a worse case of it, I don't think the experiences with the cancers have made it better or worse.

The danger of writing a memoir is that you might start to believe your own narrative. You know, that perhaps cancer challenges and changes the fundamental self in profound ways and that perhaps the writing of a memoir reveals that self. I now have two incurable, if treatable, cancers. I'll die with them, if not from one or the other. What I think now is that illness is not an identity, not a self, as much time and energy as it may take away from any particular day. We like to think that the self is unique, that our own inner being is more uniquely *us* than our outer presentation, that walk, that way of holding our head that makes each of us instantly recognizable from a distance. Illness, in the larger sense of mortality, is an inescapable shared trait among all living creatures, and we humans know about it, whether or not we want to talk about it.

So my cancer is not my self but without my cancer I would in a sense still be looking harder for my self. I, my self, am at peace with mortality, even if we are not the best of friends; it's always here with me. Before my encounters with cancer, I think, mortality was a stranger patiently waiting for an inevitable appointment with my self. Heather pointed out on reading this chapter that I am unconsciously echoing Emily Dickinson here. I'm thinking now that I owe Dickinson a long careful reading. In any case, now mortality and I know each other. We, my self and my mortality, are like adjacent pieces of a jigsaw puzzle, securely and comfortably locked together in a picture left out in the sun, bound to gradually fade and disappear together.

There is no yesterday; there is no tomorrow; there is only the infinite now. And it appears to me that the Buddha is always laughing.

Heather Responds to "Epilogue"

Well. I am somewhat uncomfortable having the last personal word here before "Acknowledgments." So I'll just make a few observations on where we've been and where we are and what we may have learned along the way. First, we are hardly special. Since Don's initial cancer diagnosis, I've learned there's almost no one we know who hasn't experienced a serious illness firsthand or lost a friend or family member to cancer or something just as bad. Most of my women friends who are older than I am have lost their husbands to cancer. And yet when you're going through the experience it's hard not to feel singled out by fate. The only thing that probably sets us apart from some others is that we choose to write about it.

What else have we learned? Primarily, how hard it is to navigate the healthcare system with a serious illness or two. The amount of research and questioning it takes to become reasonably knowledgeable about disease and treatment options, billing and insurance, and procedures is staggering and the information difficult to process. I don't know how people who don't do research for a living keep from being overwhelmed. I don't know how people manage who aren't, like me, pleasantly pushy (and occasionally fierce) administrators who regularly have to squeeze information out of professionals and bureaucrats in order to get things done. And sometimes, if rarely, recognize and challenge apparent incompetence.

But the hardest thing for me to deal with has been what I don't know or understand. Watching someone you love suffer in terrible pain when no one can figure out a cause that would then lead to a solution was awful for me—worse than Don's cancer diagnosis. I might compare it to how I feel when I see him suffer through a bad bout with depression: I feel bad for him but can't understand what he's going through, except abstractly. And I can't help him. Same with anxiety attacks, though I find those easier to understand; but I have a hard time dealing with such irrational thinking coming from someone who is one of the smartest people I know. What is the commonality? Lack of control, I think.

Then there's making peace with mortality, as Don describes it. Notice he doesn't say "death" or "dying," unlike Dickinson, who basically says, "Hey, thanks, Death." Of course, she believed in immortality and thought that was where she was heading. And it was much harder to practice denial of death, perhaps, in the nineteenth century, when it was so much a part of everyday life. I think I began to make peace with Death the moment my father died, with me holding his hand and telling him it was all right and time to let go and move on. His death made dying seem not so scary anymore. Now *suffering*—that's another story.

Let's talk about that "everyday life." Once the initial shock of each diagnosis was past, that's what took over each time. However profound the experience may seem at first (and it sucks the air out of the room, as Don has suggested), the quotidian, the day-to-day, takes over. Our *demandos* (cats and dog) want their food on schedule and preferably fifteen minutes early. No excuses. Dishwashers require emptying and refrigerators need fixing. Bills are payable on receipt, right? Elections come and go and occupy your attention for a time. People are unflaggingly kind, or they are the opposite. Does the self change then? That's one of Don's preoccupations. Whatever that means. I say no. What probably changes is the story you construct about your self. But that is always a work in progress anyway. And we are always inclined to believe in our own narrative.

Notes
1. "Diagnosing Carcinoid Tumors and Carcinoid Syndrome."

Bibliography

"AbbVie Inc Imbruvica, Magical Molecule for Rare Disease." *BidnessEtc,* 2016. Accessed September 27, 2017. web.archive.org/web/20160828130651/www. bidnessetc.com/72684-abbvie-imbruvica-magical-molecule-rare-diseases/.

"Ain't Nobody Got Time for That." *Urban Dictionary,* 2017. Accessed September 26, 2017. www.urbandictionary.com/define.php?term=Ain%27t+nobody+got+time+ for+that.

Alsop, Stewart. *Stay of Execution: A Sort of Memoir.* Philadelphia: J. B. Lippincott, 1973.

Angell, Marcia. *The Truth About the Drug Companies: How They Deceive Us and What to Do About It.* New York: Random House, 2005.

Angwin, Julia. *Dragnet Nation: A Quest for Privacy, Security, and Freedom in a World of Relentless Surveillance.* New York: Henry Holt, 2014.

"AstraZeneca Completes Transaction for Majority Equity Stake Investment in Acerta Pharma." *BiogenerationVentures,* 2016. Accessed September 27, 2017. www.biogenerationventures.com/astrazeneca-completes-transaction-for -majority-equity-stake-investment-in-acerta-pharma/_389_n__32_NL_103.

Awan, Farrukh T. "Cure for CLL?" *Blood* 127, no. 274 (2016). Accessed September 26, 2017. www.bloodjournal.org/content/127/3/274?sso-checked=true.

Baum, Joel A., and Rafael Antonio Ching Companioni. "Meckel Diverticulum." *Merck Manual,* 2017. Accessed October 1, 2017. www.merckmanuals.com/ professional/gastrointestinal-disorders/diverticular-disease/meckel -diverticulum.

Becker, Ernest. *The Denial of Death.* New York: Free Press, 1973.

"Bone Marrow and Stem Cell Transplant for Chronic Lymphocytic Leukaemia (CLL)." London: Cancer Research UK, 2015. Accessed September 26, 2017. www. cancerresearchuk.org/about-cancer/type/cll/treatment/bone-marrow-and -stem-cell-transplant-for-chronic-lymphocytic-leukaemia.

Boot, Max. "Rebrand It However You Want, but Afghanistan Is Still at War." *Los Angeles Times,* September 28, 2016. Accessed September 26, 2017. www.latimes. com/nation/la-oe-boot-afghanistan-war-end-20141230-story.html.

Broderick, Jason M. "Cheson Highlights Choices in Frontline CLL Care." *OncLive,* September 1, 2016. Accessed September 27, 2017. www.onclive.com/web -exclusives/cheson-highlights-choices-in-frontline-cll-care.

"Brownies by Fairytale." Fairytale Brownies, 2017. Accessed October 1, 2017. www. brownies.com/.

Burke, Darla. "Meckel's Diverticulum." *Healthline,* 2017. Accessed October 1, 2017. www.healthline.com/health/meckels-diverticulum#Symptoms2.

"Cancer Stat Fact Sheets: Chronic Lymphocytic Leukemia (CLL)." NIH: National Cancer Institute, 2017. Accessed September 27, 2017. seer.cancer.gov/statfacts/html/clyl.html.

Carnie, Andrew. *Syntax A Generative Introduction.* 3rd ed. Malden, MA: Blackwell, 2013.

Castle, Erik P. "Pomegranate Juice: A Cure for Prostate Cancer." Mayo Clinic, 2017. Accessed October 1,2017. www.mayoclinic.org/diseases-conditions/prostate-cancer/expert-answers/pomegranate-juice/faq-20058204.

Chemotherapy and You: Support for People with Cancer. National Cancer Institute, June 2011. Accessed September 25, 2017. www.cancer.gov/publications/patient-education/chemo-and-you.

"Chemotherapy for Chronic Lymphocytic Leukemia." Atlanta: American Cancer Society, 2016. Accessed September 24, 2017. www.cancer.org/cancer/leukemia-chroniclymphocyticcll/detailedguide/leukemia-chronic-lymphocytic-treating-chemotherapy.

Chen, Yi-Bin. "WBC Count." *MedLinePlus.* Washington, DC: National Institutes of Health, 2017. Accessed September 22, 2017. medlineplus.gov/ency/article/003643.htm.

Chozick, Amy. "Obama Addresses Afghan War's End on Christmas Visit." *New York Times,* December 25, 2014. Accessed September 26, 2017. www.nytimes.com/2014/12/26/us/obama-addresses-afghan-wars-end-on-christmas-visit.html.

ChucklenutShirts.com. Accessed September 24, 2017. www.cafepress.com/chucklenut/2619770.

"Clinical Trial Phases." NIH: U.S. National Library of Medicine, 2008. Accessed September 26, 2017. web.archive.org/web/20160918002334/www.nlm.nih.gov/services/ctphases.html.

Coffey, Brendan. "Scientology Donor Becomes a Billionaire with Cancer Drug." *Bloomberg,* January 29, 2013. Accessed September 26, 2017. web.archive.org/web/20130204042738/www.bloomberg.com/news/2013-01-29/scientology-donor-becomes-a-billionaire-with-cancer-drug.html.

Corner, Ben. "Ibrutinib's Breakthrough to Market." PharmExec.com, December 25, 2013. Accessed September 26, 2017. blog.pharmexec.com/2013/11/25/ibrutinibs-breakthrough-to-market/.

"Costs of War: Economic Costs." Brown University Watson Institute, 2016. Accessed September 26, 2017. watson.brown.edu/costsofwar/costs/economic.

Davies, Mark. *The Corpus of Contemporary American English.* Provo: Brigham Young University, 2017

"Diagnosing Carcinoid Tumors and Carcinoid Syndrome." Novartis Oncology, 2017. Accessed September 29, 2017. www.carcinoid.com/health-care-professional/

carcinoid-biochemical-testing.jsp?usertrack.filter_applied=true&NovaId
=2935377057500132198.

Dumper, Jaymi, et al. "Complications of Meckel's Diverticula in Adults." *Cancer Journal of Surgery* 49, no. 5 (2006). Accessed October 1, 2017. www.ncbi.nlm.nih. gov/pmc/articles/PMC3207587/.

Editors of AARP. "Why Drugs Cost So Much." *AARP Bulletin* 58, no. 4 (2017): 16-24.

The Fabric of the Cosmos: Universe or Multiverse. PBS, 2011. Accessed September 28, 2017. www.pbs.org/wgbh/nova/physics/fabric-of-cosmos.html#fabric -multiverse.

"FCR Chemotherapy." Macmillan Cancer Support, 2016. Accessed September 24, 2017. www.macmillan.org.uk/cancerinformation/cancertreatment/ treatmenttypes/chemotherapy/combinationregimen/fcr.aspx.

"Fevers: When Cancer Becomes an Emergency." Cleveland Clinic, 2014. Accessed September 24, 2017. health.clevelandclinic.org/2014/02/fevers-when-cancer -becomes-an-emergency/.

Fikes, Bradley J. "New Approaches to Starving Cancers." *San Diego Union-Tribune,* June 25, 2015. Accessed October 1, 2017. www.sandiegouniontribune.com/ business/biotech/sdut-autophagy-cancer-shaw-cosford-2015jun25-htmlstory. html.

Folger, Tim. "Science's Alternative to an Intelligent Creator: The Multiverse Theory." *Discover,* December 2008. Accessed September 28, 2017. discovermagazine.com/2008/dec/10-sciences-alternative-to-an-intelligent -creator.

Gawande, Atul. *Being Mortal: Medicine and What Matters in the End.* New York: Metropolitan Books, 2014.

Gersten, Todd. "Bone Marrow Aspiration." *MedLinePlus.* Washington, DC: National Institutes of Health, 2016. Accessed September 23, 2017. medlineplus.gov/ency/ article/003658.htm.

Gooch, Brad. *Flannery: A Life of Flannery O'Connor.* New York: Little, Brown, 2009.

Greenwald, David. "Sedation: Propofol Versus Conscious Sedation; Who Should Administer It?" GastroHep.com, May 3, 2006. Accessed September 28, 2017. www.gastrohep.com/freespeech/freespeech.asp?id=101.

Hadhazy, Adam. "Think Twice: How the Gut's 'Second Brain' Influences Mood and Well-Being," *Scientific American,* February 12, 2010. Accessed October 1, 2017. www.scientificaamerican.com/article/gut-second-brain/.

Harris, Sam. *Waking Up: A Guide to Spirituality Without Religion.* New York: Simon & Schuster, 2014.

Heidegger, Martin. *Being and Time.* Translated by John Macquarrie and Edward Robinson. New York: Harper & Row, 1962.

———. *An Introduction to Metaphysics.* Translated by Ralph Manheim. New Haven: Yale University Press, 1959.

Herper, Matthew. "A Lucky Drug Made Pharmacyclics' Robert Duggan a Billionaire, Will Long-Term Success Follow?" *Forbes,* April 16, 2014. Accessed September 30, 2017. www.forbes.com/sites/matthewherper/2014/04/16/a-lucky-drug-made-pharmacyclics-robert-duggan-a-billionaire-will-long-term-success-follow/#25a81b1440ed.

Hillmen, Peter. "Richter's Syndrome: CLL Taking a Turn for the Worse." *Oncology,* December 19, 2012. Accessed September 25, 2017. www.cancernetwork.com/articles/richters-syndrome-cll-taking-turn-worse.

"Hodgkin Lymphoma." Atlanta: American Cancer Society, 2017. Accessed September 23, 2017. www.cancer.org/cancer/hodgkin-lymphoma.html.

Hooper, Rowan. "Multiverse Me: Should I Care About My Other Selves?" *New Scientist,* September 24, 2014. Accessed September 25, 2017. www-newscientist-com.unr.idm.oclc.org/article/mg22329880-400-multiverse-me-should-i-care-about-my-other-selves/.

Iliades, Chris. "What a High PSA Level Means if It's Not Prostate Cancer." *Everyday Health,* 2017. Accessed September 27, 2017. www.everydayhealth.com/prostate-cancer/non-cancerous-reasons-your-psa-levels-are-high.aspx.

"Index." *Harper's,* September 2016, 9.

Inman, Matthew. "How to Perfectly Load a Dishwasher." *The Oatmeal,* 2016. Accessed 09/26/2017. theoatmeal.com/comics/dishwasher.

"Is Long-Term Remission with FCR a Cure?" Patient Power, 2013. Accessed September 27, 2017. www.patientpower.info/video/is-long-term-cll-remission-with-fcr-a-cure.

Jain, Nitin. "New Developments in Richter Syndrome." *Clinical Advances in Hematology & Oncology* 13, no. 4 (2015). Accessed September 25, 2017. www.hematologyandoncology.net/index.php/archives/april-2015/new-developments-in-richter-syndrome/.

Jain, Nitin, and Susan O'Brien. "Chronic Lymphocytic Leukemia with Deletion 17p: Emerging Treatment Options." *Oncology,* November 16, 2012. Accessed September 25, 2017. www.cancernetwork.com/chronic-lymphocytic-leukemia/chronic-lymphocytic-leukemia-deletion-17p-emerging-treatment-options.

Johnson, George. *The Cancer Chronicles: Unlocking Medicine's Deepest Mystery.* New York: Vintage Books, 2013.

Kounang, Nadia. "Opioid Addiction Rates Continue to Skyrocket." *CNN,* June 29, 2017. Accessed September 29, 2017. www.cnn.com/2017/06/29/health/opioid-addiction-rates-increase-500/index.html.

Kriss, Sam. "The Multiverse Idea Is Rotting Culture." *Atlantic,* August 29, 2016. Accessed September 28, 2017. www.theatlantic.com/science/archive/2016/08/the-multiverse-as-imagination-killer/497417/.

Larkin, Philip. "Aubade." *Times Literary Supplement* (London), December 23, 1977, 1491.

"Leukaemia: Reactions to the Diagnosis." healthtalk.org. Oxford: University of Oxford, 2015. Accessed September 23, 2017. www.healthtalk.org/peoples -experiences/cancer/leukaemia/reactions-diagnosis.

Leung, Rebecca. "Prescriptions and Profit: Why Are Americans Paying More for Medication?" *CBS News*, March 12, 2004. Accessed September 26, 2017. www. cbsnews.com/news/prescriptions-and-profit-12-03-2004/.

"Living Through Rotator Cuff Injury and Surgery." *Virginian-Pilot* (Norfolk, VA), July 31, 2013. Accessed September 29, 2017. pilotonline.com/life/fitness/quick -tips-for-wellness/living-through-rotator-cuff-injury-and-surgery/article _55f3fd11-e9cd-5fb1-8616-577da1633a96.html.

McRaney, David. "The Backfire Effect." *You Are Not So Smart: A Celebration of Self Delusion*, October 1, 2017. Accessed September 26, 2017. youarenotsosmart.com/ 2011/06/10/the-backfire-effect/.

Mooney, Chris. "The Science of Why We Don't Believe Science: How Our Brains Fool Us on Climate, Creationism, and the Vaccine-Autism Link." *Mother Jones*, May–June 2011. Accessed October 1, 2017. www.motherjones.com/politics/2011/ 03/denial-science-chris-mooney.

The New Oxford Annotated Bible. 4th ed. Oxford: Oxford University Press, 2010.

O'Connor, Flannery. *Collected Works*. New York: Library of America, 1988.

"Oprah's Favorite Pomegranate Martini Recipe." Drinks Mixer, 2017. Accessed October 1, 2017. www.drinksmixer.com/drink12149.html.

Oxford English Dictionary. Oxford: Oxford University Press, 2017. Accessed online September 23, 2017

Pausch, Randy. "Randy Pausch's Last Lecture." Carnegie Mellon University, 2007. Accessed September 26, 2017. www.cmu.edu/randyslecture/.

Pausch, Randy, and Jeffrey Zaslow. *The Last Lecture*. New York: Hyperion Books, 2008.

"Pharmaceutical Industry." World Health Organization, 2016. Accessed September 26, 2016, from WaybackMachine Internet Archive. web.archive.org/web/ 20160108031146/www.who.int/trade/glossary/story073/en/.

"Pharmaceuticals." Global Regulatory Services, 2016. Accessed September 26, 2017. web.archive.org/web/20160903110331/www.globalregulatoryservices.com/ industry-sectors/pharmaceuticals-general.

"Phase III Study Strengthens Support of Ibrutinib as Second-Line Therapy for CLL and SLL." European Society for Medical Oncology, 2014. Accessed September 26, 2017. www.esmo.org/Oncology-News/Phase-III-Study-Strengthens-Support -of-Ibrutinib-as-Second-line-Therapy-for-CLL-and-SLL.

Plato. *The Republic of Plato*. Translated by Francis MacDonald Cornford. New York: Oxford University Press, 1941.

"Policy Basics: Where Do Our Federal Tax Dollars Go?" Washington, DC: Center on Budget and Policy Priorities, 2016. Accessed September 26, 2017. www.cbpp.org/

research/federal-budget/policy-basics-where-do-our-federal-tax-dollars-go?fa
=view&id=1258.

Pollock, Rufus. "Strong Words from WHO on Pharma Industry." rufuspollock.org,
2016. Accessed September 26, 2017. rufuspollock.org/2016/05/29/strong-words
-from-who-on-pharma-industry/.

"Priapism: Overview." Mayo Clinic, 2017. Accessed September 23, 2017. www.
mayoclinic.org/diseases-conditions/priapism/home/ovc-20208946.

"Priapism: Symptoms and Causes." Mayo Clinic, 2017. Accessed September 23, 2017.
www.mayoclinic.org/diseases-conditions/priapism/symptoms-causes/dxc
-20208950.

"Propofol Side Effects." Drugs.com, 2017. Accessed September 23, 2016. www.drugs.
com/sfx/propofol-side-effects.html.

"Prostate-Specific Antigen (PSA) Test." NIH: National Cancer Institute, 2017.
Accessed October 1, 2017. www.cancer.gov/types/prostate/psa-fact-sheet.

Rabinowitz, Simon S. "Pediatric Meckel Diverticulum." Medscape, 2016. Accessed
October 1, 2017. emedicine.medscape.com/article/931229-overview.

"Rituxan." RxList, 2016. Accessed September 25, 2017. www.rxlist.com/rituxan
-side-effects-drug-center.htm.

Roach, Mary. Stiff: The Curious Lives of Human Cadavers. New York: Norton, 2003.

"Robert Duggan." Forbes: The World's Billionaires, 2016. Accessed September 27, 2017.
web.archive.org/web/20160919084254/www.forbes.com/profile/robert
-duggan.

Schumacher, Julie. Dear Committee Members. New York: Anchor, 2015.

Senthilkumaran, Subramanian, et al. "Propofol and Priapism." Indian Journal of
Pharmacology 42, no. 4 (2010): 238–39. Accessed September 23, 2017. www.ncbi.
nlm.nih.gov/pmc/articles/PMC2941615/.

Shaffer, Anita T. "Next-Generation BTK Inhibitor Taking on Ibrutinib in CLL."
OncLive, 2015. Accessed September 27, 2017. www.onclive.com/conference
-coverage/ash-2015/next-generation-btk-inhibitor-taking-on-ibrutinib-in-cll.

Shaywitz, David. "The Wild Story Behind a Promising Experimental Cancer Drug."
Forbes, April 5, 2013. Accessed September 26, 2016. www.forbes.com/sites/
davidshaywitz/2013/04/05/the-wild-story-behind-a-promising-experimental
-cancer-drug/.

Sidner, Sara. "Fentanyl: The Powerful Opioid That Killed Prince." CNN, June 3, 2016.
Accessed September 29, 2017. www.cnn.com/2016/05/10/health/fentanyl-new
-heroin-deadlier/index.html.

Understanding CLL/SLL: A Guide for Patients, Survivors, and Loved Ones. Lymphoma
Research Foundation, 2010. Accessed September 25, 2017. www.lymphoma.org/
atf/cf/%7Baaf3b4e5-2c43-404c-afe5-fd903c87b254%7D/CLL_BOOK12.10.PDF.

Understanding CLL/SLL: A Guide for Patients, Survivors, and Loved Ones. New York:
Lymphoma Research Foundation, 2016. Accessed September 22, 2017. www.
lymphoma.org (see under "Learn," "Booklets/Fact Sheets," "CLL/SLL").

VICE *Special Report: Killing Cancer,* 2015. Accessed October 1, 2017. www.youtube. com/watch?v=j8Xky-UvMyA&list=ELLtV9LYXF9xYGzMWVQguahw.

Vilenkin, Alexander, and Max Tegmark. "The Case for Parallel Universes: Why the Multiverse, Crazy as It Sounds, Is a Solid Scientific Idea." *Scientific American,* July 19, 2011. Accessed September 28, 2017. www.scientificamerican.com/ article/multiverse-the-case-for-parallel-universe/.

Walker, Joseph. "Patients Struggle with High Drug Prices." *Wall Street Journal,* December 31, 2015. Accessed September 27, 2017. web.archive.org/web/ 20151231123027/www.wsj.com/articles/patients-struggle-with-high-drug-prices -1451557981.

"What Are the 5-10 Most Interesting Facts About the Pharmaceuticals Industry?" askwonder.com. Accessed September 26, 2017. askwonder.com/q/what -are-the-5-10-most-interesting-facts-about-the-pharmaceuticals-industry -56f1acf547e9241a00a3ae80.

"What Causes Lymphoma?" LymphomaInfo.net, 2016. Accessed September 23, 2016. www.lymphomainfo.net/lymphoma/causes.html.

"What Happens After Treatment for Chronic Lymphocytic Leukemia." Atlanta: American Cancer Society, 2016. Accessed September 22, 2017. www.cancer.org/ cancer/leukemia-chroniclymphocyticcll/detailedguide/leukemia-chronic -lymphocytic-after-follow-up.

"What Is Chronic Lymphocytic Leukemia?" Atlanta: American Cancer Society, 2017. Accessed September 22, 2017. www.cancer.org/cancer/leukemia -chroniclymphocyticcll/detailedguide/leukemia-chronic-lymphocytic-what -is-cll.

"What Is Prostatitis?" *WebMD,* 2017. Accessed September 27, 2017. www.webmd. com/men/guide/prostatitis.

Whitman, Walt. *Leaves of Grass,* 1892. Accessed July 2, 2017. www.gutenberg.org/ files/1322/1322-h/1322-h.htm.

Wright, Lawrence. *Going Clear: Scientology, Hollywood, and the Prison of Belief.* New York: Vintage, 2013.

Acknowledgments

I STARTED WRITING about my experience with cancer just after my diagnosis and continued to write through chemotherapy and after. I shared many of my thoughts and experiences in both blog and paper forms with friends and others. The encouragement and support I received from those incredibly kind and sympathetic readers were crucial to both my psychological well-being and my ability to continue to write through my treatment and recovery.

Because I am writing this part of the book alone, I have to thank my lovely brilliant wife Heather first. I am not at all sure I would have survived if not for her.

There are too many close friends to thank for their support individually, as you might expect after having read this account. Those whose help to Heather and me was indispensable include Jack Alfonso, Cami Allen, Charlotte Altamirano, David Barrow, Joy Batchelor, Brooke Bentley, Kathy Boardman, Phil Boardman, Tiffany Threatt Bourelle, Sharon Brush, Stacy Burton, Christina Camarena, Scott Casper, Ian Clayton, Christopher Coake, Amelia Currier, Philip Davis, Patricia Davis, Shay Daylami, Jane Detweiler, Melanie Duckworth, Dennis Dworkin, Sara Elliott, David Fenimore, Victoria Follette, Rebecca Fraga, Valerie Fridland, Jim Giles, Wanda Giles, Ibis Gomez-Vega, Amanda Hardy, Dolores Hardy, Erin Hardy, John Hardy, Oma Hardy, Robert Hardy, Tammy Hardy, Jen Hendrickson, Thomas Hertweck, Vicky Hines, Ann Keniston, Lauren Kilpatrick, Kat Lambrecht, Meredith Larson, Stephanie Lauer, Dor Macdonald, Chris MacMahon, Ashley Marshall, Elizabeth Preston, Susan Raeder, Eric Rasmussen, Kathy Ray, Ron Ray, Debra Richtmeyer, Janine Scancarelli, Karen L. Parr Schaeffer,

Bob Self, Lois Self, Susan Smith, Roxie Taft, Karen Vogel, and Lynne Waldeland.

Our editor, Justin Race, has been personally and professionally helpful in ways that only a good friend and great editor can be. Thanks to Stacy Burton for her suggestions on the final draft of the manuscript and how to respond to the very helpful external reviews. Many thanks also to Robin DuBlanc for excellent copy-editing work and numerous suggestions that improved the book.

Finally, I must acknowledge the real heroes of the book: all my nurses and doctors, anonymously presented with both love and gratitude throughout this account. You know who you are, and I hope you remember, as I do, our shared laughter, and I hope this book reminds you of your many kindnesses to Heather and me.

About the Authors

DON HARDY received a PhD in linguistics from Rice University. He taught linguistics at the University of North Texas, Northern Illinois University, Colorado State University, and the University of Nevada, Reno, where he is now professor emeritus. His research areas included corpus linguistics and stylistics. He was a 2000 winner of the Northern Illinois University Excellence in Undergraduate Teaching Award. At UNR Hardy won the Alan Bible Teaching Excellence Award, 2014, and the F. Donald Tibbetts Distinguished Teacher Award, 2016. His books *Narrating Knowledge in Flannery O'Connor's Fiction* (2003) and *The Body in Flannery O'Connor's Fiction: Computational Technique and Linguistic Voice* (2007) were published by the University of South Carolina Press. In his retirement, he writes, reads, and gives mostly unsolicited advice to his younger friends.

HEATHER HARDY was born in Houston, Texas, and graduated there from Rice University. After receiving her PhD in linguistics from UCLA in 1979, she taught linguistics at a number of universities, including the University of North Texas and Northern Illinois University. From 2003 to 2005 she served as dean of the College of Liberal Arts at Colorado State University. In 2005 she was hired by the University of Nevada, Reno, where she served as dean of liberal arts and for a time as interim executive vice president and provost before her retirement in 2015. She is happily retired and living in Reno with her husband, two cats, and a dog.